EXTRAPERITONEAL
LAPAROSCOPIC SURGERY

To Dominic, Victoria, Sacha and Harriet

Extraperitoneal Laparoscopic Surgery

EDITED BY

Christopher G. Eden MS FRCS (Urol)

Senior Registrar in Urology
Guy's and St Thomas' Hospitals
London, UK

FOREWORD BY

J. E. A. Wickham

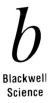

Blackwell
Science

© 1997 by
Blackwell Science Ltd
Editorial Offices:
Osney Mead, Oxford OX2 0EL
25 John Street, London WC1N 2BL
23 Ainslie Place, Edinburgh EH3 6AJ
350 Main Street, Malden
    MA 02148 5018, USA
54 University Street, Carlton
    Victoria 3053, Australia

Other Editorial Offices:
Blackwell Wissenschafts-Verlag GmbH
Kurfürstendamm 57
10707 Berlin, Germany

Blackwell Science KK
MG Kodenmacho Building
7–10 Kodenmacho Nihombashi
Chuo-ku, Tokyo 104, Japan

First published 1997

The Blackwell Science logo is a
trade mark of Blackwell Science Ltd,
registered at the United Kingdom
Trade Marks Registry

A catalogue record for this title is
available from the British Library

ISBN 0-86542-623-6

Library of Congress
Cataloging-in-publication Data

Extraperitoneal laparoscopic surgery/
    edited by Christopher G. Eden;
    foreword by J.E.A. Wickham.
        p.   cm.
    Includes bibliographical references
    and index.
    ISBN 0-86542-623-6
    1. Retroperitoneum—Endoscopic
    surgery.
    I. Eden, Christopher G.
    [DNLM: 1. Surgery, Laparoscopic—
    methods.
    WO 500 E96 1997]
RD540.E98   1997
617′.05—dc21
DNLM/DLC
for Library of Congress   96-50088
                                           CIP

Set by Setrite Typesetters, Hong Kong
Printed and bound in France by
Imprimerie Pollina SA, Luçon

DISTRIBUTORS

Marston Book Services Ltd
PO Box 269
Abingdon, Oxon OX14 4YN
(*Orders*: Tel: 01235 465500
            Fax: 01235 465555)

USA
Blackwell Science, Inc.
Commerce Place
350 Main Street
Malden, MA 02148 5018
(*Orders*: Tel: 800 759 6102
                    617 388 8250
            Fax: 617 388 8255)

Canada
Copp Clark Professional
200 Adelaide St West, 3rd Floor
Toronto, Ontario M5H 1W7
(*Orders*: Tel: 416 597-1616
                    800 815-9417
            Fax: 416 597-1617)

Australia
Blackwell Science Pty Ltd
54 University Street
Carlton, Victoria 3053
(*Orders*: Tel: 3 9347 0300
            Fax: 3 9347 5001)

Contents

List of contributors

Taha A. Abdel-Meguid MB BS MS
Fellow in Urology, Thomas Jefferson University, Philadelphia, USA and Assistant Lecturer in Urology, Minia University Hospital, Minia, Egypt

Samuel M. Andrews MA MS FRCS
Specialist Registrar in Vascular Surgery, St Thomas' Hospital, London, UK

Joris J. G. Bannenberg MD
Department of Surgery/Surgical Research, Academic Medical Centre, University of Amsterdam, The Netherlands

Roelof U. Boelhouwer MD PhD
Consultant Surgeon, Ikazia Hospital, Rotterdam, and the Department of Surgery, Erasmus University Medical School, Rotterdam, The Netherlands

Christopher G. Eden MS FRCS (Urol)
Senior Registrar in Urology, Guy's and St Thomas' Hospitals, London, UK

Durga D. Gaur MS FRCS
Consultant Urological Surgeon, Associate Professor of Urology and Honorary Consultant to the Armed Forces, Bombay Hospital Institute of Medical Sciences, Bombay, India

Leonard G. Gomella MD
Bernard W. Godwin Jr. Associate Professor of Prostate Cancer, Department of Urology, Thomas Jefferson University, Philadelphia, USA

Robert J. S. Hawthorn MD MRCOG
Consultant Obstetrician and Gynaecologist, and Honorary Senior Lecturer, Department of Gynaecology, Southern General Hospital, Glasgow, UK

Pierre Hourlay MD
Abdominal Surgeon, Salvatorziekenhuis Surgery, Hasselt, Belgium

Alberto Mandressi MD
Head of Urological Operative Unit, Busto Arsizio Hospital, Busto Arsizio (VA), Italy

Dirk W. Meijer MD PhD MSc
Department of Surgery/Surgical Research, Academic Medical Centre, University of Amsterdam, The Netherlands

Bart M. P. Rademaker MD PhD
Staff Anesthesiologist and Intensivist, Department of Anesthesiology and Intensive Care, Academic Medical Centre, Amsterdam, The Netherlands

Jens J. Rassweiler MD
*Professor and Chief of Urology, Chefarzt, Urologische Klinik, Stadtisches
Krankenhaus Heilbronn, Am Gesundbrunnen, 74078 Heilbronn, Germany*

Cornelius J. van Steensel MD PhD
*Consultant Surgeon, Ikazia Hospital, Rotterdam, and the Department of
Surgery, Erasmus University Medical School, Rotterdam, The Netherlands*

Foreword

In the mid 1970s techniques of open intra-renal surgery for the treatment of renal stones were being rapidly refined. At that time it seemed to me that conventional therapy for the management of ureteric calculus disease was quite incongruous.

To remove a 5-mm stone from the upper or mid ureter a ludicrously large incision was required. Access to the ureter had been classically a retroperitoneal approach and I attempted to reduce this trauma of access by utilizing a mini-lumbotomy incision requiring little muscular disruption. The lessening of muscular damage paid off and patients were able to leave hospital in 48 hours instead of 1 week and experienced much less post-operative morbidity.

I was still not satisfied that the operative damage was consistent with the size of the lesion dealt with, and I looked for another method whereby these ureteric stones could be accessed without significant damage to the abdominal wall.

In 1975 I felt it would be worthwhile to attempt to image the ureter from outside endoscopically. To obtain access transperitoneally appeared significantly invasive and I therefore felt it might be worthwhile to attempt a retroperitoneal approach. To do this it was obviously necessary to distend the retroperitoneal space with either fluid or gas to obtain adequate visualization and, following initial experimental work on the pig, gas distension appeared to be the most useful technique. I was interested to find that in the pig, retroperitoneal gas distension produced an excellent view of the lower pole of the kidney, renal pelvis and the ureter. The animals appeared to experience few ill effects from this technique and in 1975 I performed the first retroperitoneal insufflation for the treatment of an upper ureteric calculus in a human. Instrumentation was by an operating laparoscope inserted through a 10-mm port with an ancillary instrument passed through a 5-mm port after Veress needle insufflation in the retroperitoneum. The retroperitoneum was distended with approximately 2 litres of CO_2. Visualization and distension was not as good as that obtained in the animals. The ureter was nevertheless identified and incised over the calculus which then dropped into the retroperitoneal space and was retrieved. The ureter was not sutured and a drain was inserted. The patient made a rapid recovery, with negligible urinary leakage. The technique was, however, very difficult and ureteric identification was time-consuming.

Over the next year or two I performed four further ureterolithotomy operations, succeeding in two and failing in two.

In 1979 I performed the first elective percutaneous endoscopic nephro-lithotomy and thereafter went intraluminal and the retroperitoneal approach was abandoned. I always felt that this method should be exploited further and fully believed that a retroperitoneal nephrectomy was a significant possibility and this was subsequently demonstrated by Ralph Clayman in the USA and Jens Rassweiler in Europe.

I have also been very impressed by the developments that have occurred in the last few years, particularly by the work of Durga Gaur with balloon dis-tension and exploitation of the retroperitoneum for the treatment of various conditions.

To anyone who has had experience of abdominal surgery over many years it must be obvious that patients make much faster post-operative progress and with less morbidity when the peritoneal cavity or the abdominal wall is not seriously transgressed. The retroperitoneal approach to a number of pathologies must surely be commended for this factor alone.

Christopher Eden is to be commended for assembling such a talented col-lection of authorities to review this increasingly important area of surgery. There is always much more to be done and the retroperitoneal approach will, I am sure, be increasingly refined over the next decade. Operations of this nature require a much greater degree of skill than the rather unthinking meth-ods of open surgery.

In any therapy one must surely strive continually for improvement. There is always 'a better way to do it'. Retroperitoneal endoscopic surgery is another step along this path to increasingly less traumatic patient management, and I commend this volume to those physicians who are motivated to minimize the effects of operative trauma in any situation.

J. E. A. Wickham

Preface

The practice of laparoscopy is changing. The days of performing a complex case laparoscopically simply to produce a case report have long since gone. It remains for the players left in the game to justify each and every aspect of the laparoscopic operations that they perform, and to prospectively record and honestly report the results of their endeavours so that Ralph Clayman's question can be answered: 'it is possible, but is it better?'

The increasing acceptance of an extraperitoneal endoscopic approach to extraperitoneal structures is a good example of such reasoned thinking, being motivated as it is by what is best for the patient, rather than what is most convenient for the surgeon (extraperitoneal laparoscopy is usually more difficult than its transperitoneal counterpart). The aim of this book is to shorten the learning curve for interested surgeons by didactic instruction. Each chapter in this book has been written by an expert, the experience of whom is unique in many cases.

It is appropriate that John Wickham, the initial proponent of extraperitoneal laparoscopy (and so much else in urology) in the 1970s, was asked to write the foreword to this book and I am honoured that he has agreed. I am also honoured by the contribution of two chapters by Durga Gaur, whose description of a balloon dissector for retroperitoneoscopy in 1992 was instrumental in resurrecting interest in this approach, from which many patients have benefited. I am also grateful for the forbearance of the various contributors in allowing me to freely edit their chapters.

C. G. Eden

1 Development

C. G. EDEN

The Greek word λαπαρα (lapara) means 'the flank'. Thus, although laparoscopy has become synonymous with peritoneoscopy, true laparoscopy is really retroperitoneal endoscopy.

The concept of retroperitoneoscopy is not a new one, combining the two techniques of peritoneoscopy and retroperitoneal pneumography [1]. The latter technique is a crude but effective imaging modality for the investigation of suspected retroperitoneal pathology (Figs 1.1 and 1.2) and, when combined with tomography, represented the best imaging technique available for the retroperitoneum before the advent of grey-scale ultrasound and computed tomography.

The past

The first attempts at retroperitoneoscopy were performed by Wickham in the late 1970s. In his classic series of cadaveric experiments he confirmed the feasibility of retroperitoneal endoscopy, but also noted that limited access and the consequent poor vision caused significant problems [2]. Following the disappointment of his initial experiments he abandoned the use of direct carbon dioxide (CO_2) insufflation and chose instead to introduce air pressurized by a sigmoidoscope bulb insufflator into the retroperitoneum via a laparoscope. This led to significantly better vision, but the resulting workspace was still relatively small and the rate of instrumental damage to the kidney was high. Despite this, in 1978 he succeeded in performing a laparoscopic extraperitoneal ureterolithotomy in three of five cases attempted (J.E.A. Wickham, personal communication).

Kaplan's study of experimental retroperitoneoscopy the following year, with preliminary nitrous oxide insufflation introduced via a pre-sacral needle and blind lateral trocar insertion in 13 dogs, showed the technique to be a safe and rapid method of examining the kidneys, upper ureters, adrenals, inferior vena cava and aorta, and of performing renal biopsy under vision [3]. The sole complication in this series was perforation of a renal vein during adrenal biopsy, resulting in the death of the animal 6 hours following the procedure.

Bay-Nielsen described a simple and successful technique for human ureterolithotomy in 1982, using digital localization of the stone and the subsequent use of a laryngoscope to display the ureter and allow removal

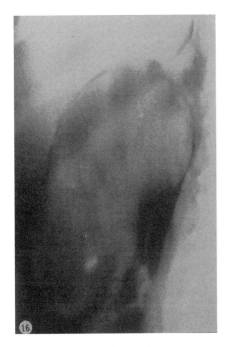

Fig. 1.1 Upper pole renal tumour demonstrated by retroperitoneal pneumography [1]. (Reproduced with permission; © 1955, American Medical Association.)

of the offending stone [4]. However, it was apparent that other retro-peritoneal structures could not be safely accessed using this technique, due to the extremely limited field of view.

In 1983 Fantoni described a technique of pelvic and medium-low retroperitoneoscopy for biopsy of retroperitoneal lymph nodes and tumours under local anaesthesia, using a mediastinoscope [5]. Following initial blind finger dissection of the retroperitoneum alongside the common iliac artery, via a small incision medial to the anterior superior iliac spine, further blunt dissection was carried out using the laparoscope. He reported no intra- or post-operative complications in the 11 operated patients.

In 1985 Clayman and co-workers reported a single case of percu-taneous retroperitoneal ureterolithotomy for an upper ureteric calculus, refractory to antegrade and retrograde manipulation [6]. The stone was located under fluoroscopic control with a needle and a guide wire passed alongside it. A percutaneous access track was then dilated over the wire, and a 30F Amplatz sheath advanced up to it. No attempt was made to produce a retroperitoneal workspace for dissection. A flexible nephro-scope was passed up to the stone as a guide and a Sachse urethrotome was used to incise the ureter over the stone, which was then retrieved. A neph-rostomy tube provided temporary urinary diversion, prior to antegrade double-pigtail stenting after 48 hours.

Weinberg and Smith performed a subtotal nephrectomy in a pig in 1988 using an endoscopic ultrasonic aspirator inserted percutaneously into the kidney under direct vision and fluoroscopic guidance through a dilated nephrostomy track [7]. The kidney had been embolized immediately pre-operatively with metal coils. The authors' concern that they were not certain of the location of the tip of the resecting aspirator at all times was confirmed by the presence of irrigation fluid in the retroperitoneum at the post-mortem examination performed immediately following surgery.

Not surprisingly, in view of the narrow margin for safety due to the limited workspace obtained during the foregoing feasibility studies, enthusiasm for retroperitoneoscopy waned. It was revived in 1992 by Gaur's description of the simple but effective technique of introducing a balloon, consisting of the amputated finger of a surgeon's glove, through a small stab incision into the retroperitoneum under direct vision, and inflating it to dissect off the peritoneum and so create a workspace [8]. Since that time, the ability to rapidly and consistently create a retroperitoneal workspace of sufficient capacity to allow safe endoscopic surgery with minimal bleeding has appealed to an increasing number of urologists (whose instinct has always been to approach the retroperitoneum from the flank) and non-urological surgeons.

The present

There is little doubt that extraperitoneal laparoscopy is usually more technically demanding than its transperitoneal counterpart. This is chiefly because the landmarks that exist in the peritoneal cavity to guide

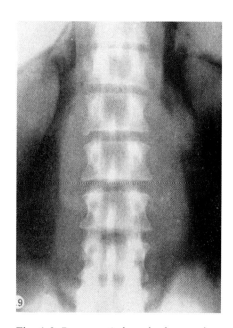

Fig. 1.2 Para-aortic lymphadenopathy demonstrated by retroperitoneal pneumography [1]. (Reproduced with permission; © 1955, American Medical Association.)

dissection are absent in the retroperitoneum but also, to a lesser extent, because the space available in which to operate is smaller, leaving less margin for error in port placement, manual dexterity and haemostasis. The advantages of not violating the peritoneal cavity unnecessarily, however, are significant for the following reasons.

1 Greater safety during access (avoiding blind Veress needle introduction and trocar insertion), surgery (avoiding diathermy injury to the bowel due to capacitance coupling, faulty insulation and direct injury) and following surgery (avoiding adhesive small-bowel obstruction and the consequent risk of ischaemia).

2 Access to the target organ, such as the kidney, is more direct (Fig. 1.3), requiring less tissue dissection, manipulation and retraction.

3 A suggestion that post-operative analgesic requirements may be lower than in patients undergoing the same procedure via the transperitoneal laparoscopic route [9,10] possibly by avoiding stimulation of peritoneal stretch receptors and nociceptors by CO_2, carbonic acid and blood.

Two studies have reported greater intra-operative CO_2 absorption during retroperitoneoscopy, compared with equivalent transperitoneal laparoscopic surgery [11,12]. These studies are of questionable clinical relevance since no adverse sequelae were noted in the retroperitoneoscopic group and since the cavity inflation pressures (15 mmHg) were unnecessarily high in this group, given that the weight of ipsilateral colon tends to maintain the retroperitoneal cavity when the patient is in the lateral position, even if the gas supply fails altogether.

Concern regarding the possibility of latex allergy [13] has persuaded some surgeons to adopt the use of a purpose-designed silicone balloon for creation of the initial extraperitoneal space, citing also the advantage of visualizing the dissection caused by the balloon in real time. The routine use of silicone balloons (Fig. 1.4), which are considerably more expensive than their readily-available latex counterparts (finger of surgical glove,

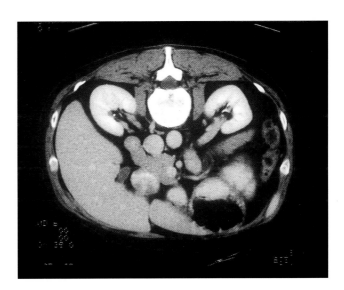

Fig. 1.3 Computed tomogram at level of second lumbar vertebra.

whole glove, condom or Helmstein balloon catheter, Fig. 1.5) is probably unjustified in terms of greater safety unless the surgical team is prepared to abandon the use of all latex products that may come into contact with the patient on a routine basis. Since the use of latex is widespread in surgery, the cost implications of avoiding latex use are so great and the consequences of anaphylaxis so potentially devastating, that it is not inconceivable that routine pre-operative testing of patients will become the norm in the foreseeable future, and will also form the basis for the exclusion of latex products.

Strong views are also held as to the relative merits and de-merits of balloon distension by either gas or saline, but to date no convincing evidence for these convictions has been advanced by either camp. In the absence of such evidence, the use of the cheapest, least messy and most readily available medium (room air) seems to make the most sense.

The future

Although comparison of complications and final outcome of laparoscopic procedures with their open surgical counterparts is essential to justify

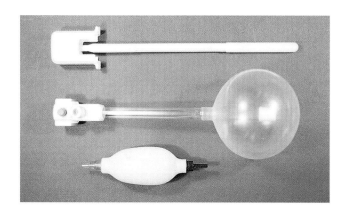

Fig. 1.4 Silicone balloon trocar (Origin Medsystems, Inc.; Menlo Park, USA; cost at time of printing was £58.06).

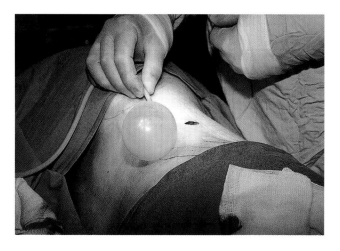

Fig. 1.5 Helmstein balloon catheter (Rusch Manufacturing (UK) Ltd, Lurgan, Northern Ireland; cost at time of printing was £25.00).

their continued use, the participation of an expert extraperitoneal laparo-scopist in a randomized clinical trial of trans- versus extraperitoneal laparoscopy might be construed as being unethical for the reasons stated above. These reasons, combined with the threat or reality of litigation, are likely to convince laparoscopists who are currently comfortable with approaching extraperitoneal organs through a transperitoneal route that there might be a better way of proceeding.

References

1 Steinbach HL, Smith DR. Extraperitoneal pneumography in diagnosis of retroperitoneal tumours. *Arch Surg* 1955; 70: 161–172.

2 Wickham JEA, Miller RA. Percutaneous renal access. In: Wickham JEA, Miller RA (eds) *Percutaneous Renal Surgery.* New York: Churchill Livingstone, 1983: 33–39.

3 Kaplan LR, Johnston GR, Hardy RM. Retroperitoneoscopy in dogs. *Gastrointest Endosc* 1979; 25: 13–15.

4 Bay-Nielsen H, Schulz A. Endoscopic retroperitoneal removal of stones from the upper half of the ureter. *Scand J Urol* 1982; 16: 227–228.

5 Fantoni PA, Mondina P, Tognoli S *et al.* Retroperitoneoscopy for biopsy of pelvic and medium-low para-aortic lymph nodes and tissues. *Int Surg* 1983; 68: 157–160.

6 Clayman RV, Preminger GM, Franklin JF, Curry T, Peters PC. Percutaneous ureterolithotomy. *J Urol* 1985; 133: 671–673.

7 Weinberg JJ, Smith AD. Percutaneous resection of the kidney: preliminary report. *J Endourol* 1988; 2: 355–359.

8 Gaur DD. Laparoscopic operative retroperitoneoscopy: use of a new device. *J Urol* 1992; 148: 1137–1139.

9 Eden CG, Murray KHA. Retroperitoneoscopic simple nephrectomy—initial experience (unpublished).

10 Clayman RV, McDougall EM, Kerbl K, Anderson K, Kavoussi LR. Laparoscopic nephrectomy: transperitoneal vs. retroperitoneal. *J Urol* 1994; 151: 342 [abstract].

11 Wolf JS Jr, Monk TG, McDougall EM, McClennan BL, Clayman RV. Factors associated with CO_2 absorption during laparoscopy. *J Urol* 1995; 153: 481 [abstract].

12 Lund O, Winfield HN, Donovan JF, Loening SA, Ping STS. Comparison of carbon dioxide (CO_2) homeostasis during intra- or extraperitoneal laparoscopic pelvic lymphadenectomy (LPLND). *J Urol* 1995; 153: 513 [abstract].

13 Hamann CP, Kick SA. What the practising urologist should know about latex allergies today. *AUA Update Series* 1994; 13: 110–115.

2

Access techniques

D. D. GAUR

A direct retroperitoneal laparoscopic approach to structures on the posterior abdominal wall is a logical option and surgeons throughout the world are familiar with this route for open surgical exploration. However, until recently the tortuous transperitoneal route was the only avenue open to the laparoscopic surgeon, due to the mostly poor results of retroperitoneoscopy in the past. The development of the balloon technique of retroperitoneoscopy by the author [1] has remarkably improved the results and has established it as the procedure of choice for the laparoscopic surgery of retroperitoneal organs.

Conventional access techniques

Both open and closed access techniques may be used to perform retroperitoneal laparoscopy.

Wickham's open technique

In 1979 Wickham described the use of a standard laparoscope and pneumoinsufflation for retroperitoneal laparoscopy via a small lumbar incision (see Chapter 1) [2].

Clayman's closed technique

In this technique, a balloon occlusion ureteral catheter with a stiff guide wire is placed cystoscopically as a preliminary procedure under fluoroscopic control [3]. The stiff guide wire helps in retroperitoneoscopic identification of the ureter. The balloon at the upper end of the catheter inflated with contrast aids its retention and fluoroscopic localization. The patient is transferred to the operating room and placed in a prone position under general anaesthesia. A Veress needle is placed below the lower pole of the kidney through the lumbar triangle under fluoroscopic control and 2 litres of carbon dioxide instilled into the retroperitoneal space. The Veress needle is replaced by a 12-mm primary port, again under fluoroscopic control. The patient can be moved to the lateral position if the retroperitoneal space is found to be less than 2 litres in the prone position.

Although Clayman and colleagues were able to perform successfully a nephrectomy using this technique, they preferred the transperitoneal route for subsequent procedures, as they found the retroperitoneal approach rather unsatisfactory [3]. However, Mandressi and colleagues still use this technique with good results [4].

The main reason for the mostly poor results of retroperitoneoscopy in the past was the inability to create a satisfactory pneumoretroperitoneum merely by insufflating through the Veress needle. This is due to the presence of tough fibroareolar septa in the retroperitoneal tissue which do not yield merely to pneumoinsufflation and require the use of some force for their disruption. The author's technique of retroperitoneoscopy [1] uses the force of an expanding balloon to break up these fibroareolar septa prior to retroperitoneoscopy to make it a simple and more readily acceptable procedure.

The author's balloon access techniques

The balloon technique of retroperitoneoscopy involves placement of an inflatable balloon in the retroperitoneal space, expansion and dissection of the space by inflating the balloon, insertion of the primary port and establishment of secondary ports under visual or digital guidance.

Advantages of the balloon technique

The technique allows safe endoscopic exploration of the entire retroperitoneum from the subdiaphragmatic region to the retropubic space. The balloon neatly dissects the retroperitoneal structures and atraumatically expands the retroperitoneal space, thereby producing a clear view of the structures and an adequate space for endoscopic manipulation. It also provides haemostasis by compressing the capillaries and venules torn during dissection [5].

The ideal balloon

The balloon should ideally be a low-pressure balloon with *ex vivo* pressures between 10 and 20mmHg. The *in vivo* balloon pressure depends upon the resistance provided by the surrounding structures but, in a virgin retroperitoneal space, this is usually not more than two to three times its *ex vivo* pressure. A low-pressure balloon is less likely to cause complete occlusion of the inferior vena cava during its inflation. It is also less likely to cause tissue damage during its expansion or following rupture if air is being used to inflate it, as it would burst before achieving high pressures [6].

The shape of the balloon is relatively unimportant as a low-pressure balloon ultimately moulds into the shape of the cavity in which it is expanding. However, an oval balloon is the logical best choice as it more closely matches the shape of the retroperitoneal space. Its superiority is also predicted by Laplace's law, which states that the tension in the wall of a hollow expandable structure is directly proportional to the product of its diameter and pressure. Thus, in a round balloon, the tension would be the same all around, while in an oval balloon it would be maximum along its long axis, which should help in the longitudinal dissection of the retroperitoneal space.

The balloon can be made from a surgical glove and a red rubber catheter [1], or a Helmstein balloon may be used [7]. However, we now prefer the commercially available Gaur balloon (Endo Exports, Bombay, India), which is an inexpensive, catheterless, low-pressure balloon and one which can be fitted directly over the nozzle of the sphygmomanometer bulb without the necessity of tying it on (Fig. 2.1).

Retroperitoneal balloon access

The balloon is placed in the retroperitoneal space using one of the three following approaches [5].
1 The lumbar approach—used for structures on the posterior abdominal wall and the upper ureter but can be extended for the exploration of the mid- and even the lower ureter.
2 The iliac approach—provides a good exposure of the ipsilateral iliopelvic retroperitoneum and is used mainly for the exploration of the pelvic ureter.
3 The suprapubic approach—useful for access to the lower abdominal, retropubic and the pelvic retroperitoneal space.

Extrafascial or subfascial placement of the balloon?

The ureter is a very important landmark during abdominal retroperitoneoscopy but, being deep to fascia transversalis, it is unlikely to be exposed if the balloon is placed in the extrafascial retroperitoneal space, unless the fascia is thin or has been torn during the initial digital dissection or due to over-inflation of the balloon. Therefore, it is preferable to place the balloon deep to the fascia transversalis. For an even better exposure of the kidney, it should be placed deep to Gerota's fascia [8].

However, in the following situations no attempt should be made to place the balloon deep to the fascia due to the increased risk of damage to the parietal peritoneum.

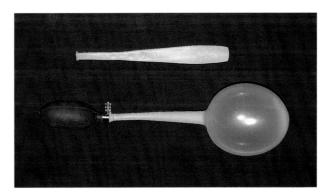

Fig. 2.1 The Gaur balloon.

1 Obese patients and patients undergoing iliac retroperitoneoscopy, as the fascia is usually thin and easily torn.
2 Patients with retroperitoneal inflammatory disease, as the tissues are oedematous, adherent and friable.
3 Patients with chronic pyelonephritis or a small high kidney, because of the technical difficulties of so doing.
4 Patients with a renal cortical cyst or malignancy, for fear of rupturing the cyst and causing tumour dissemination.

Under the above circumstances, the balloon is best placed either outside Gerota's fascia or superficial to the fascia transversalis.

The mini open balloon access technique

This technique is safe, simple and efficient. It does not involve 'blind' Veress needle insertion or primary trocar puncture, or the use of fluoroscopy for gaining retroperitoneal access.

The lumbar approach

PATIENT POSITION
The anaesthetized patient is placed in the standard lateral kidney position. The patient is tilted slightly prone for a supraumbilical procedure and supine for an infraumbilical procedure.

POSITION OF THE SURGICAL TEAM AND EQUIPMENT
Transumbilical and supraumbilical procedures. See Fig. 2.2.

Infraumbilical procedures. The surgical team moves towards the head of the patient and the nurse moves to the other side for a better view of the monitor, which is moved towards the foot-end. The first assistant stands nearer the head-end of the patient for easier manipulation of the camera.

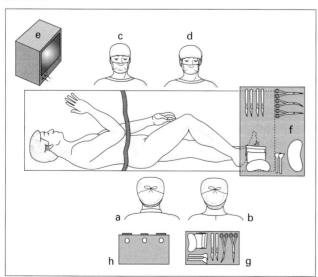

Fig. 2.2 Position of the surgical team and equipment for an umbilical or a supraumbilical retroperitoneal procedure:
a, surgeon; b, first assistant; c, second assistant; d, nurse; e, monitor; f, main instrument trolley; g, surgeon's instrument trolley; and h, diathermy machine.

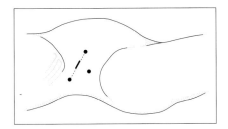

Fig. 2.3 Port sites for lumbar
retroperitoneoscopy.

PORT SITES
A subcostal kidney incision (about 20 cm long) is marked from the renal
angle to a point about 3 cm above the anterior superior spine (Fig. 2.3). A
2-cm skin incision is made along the line at its centre for insertion of the
balloon and the primary port, which approximately corresponds to the
midaxillary plane. Incisions for the secondary ports are planned at each
end of the marked line and just above the iliac crest. The three incisions
placed along the standard kidney incision line allow a neat and rapid
conversion to an open procedure if it is required.

CREATION OF THE INITIAL RETROPERITONEAL SPACE
The initial skin incision is deepened by blunt dissection with artery
forceps until the lumbodorsal fascia is reached, which can often be
appreciated by an increase in resistance. The retroperitoneal space is
entered by a short, sharp thrust of the artery forceps. The artery forceps
are pulled out with the jaws open to dilate the fascial opening, which is
further dilated with a Hegar's dilator if required. If the kidney is large or if
there is concern about accidentally damaging the peritoneum, the lumbodorsal fascia should be incised and opened up under vision, using small
retractors and a fibreoptic light.

The index finger is now introduced deep to the lumbodorsal fascia and
the retroperitoneal space dissected by gently lifting off the fascia transversalis or Gerota's fascia from the posterior abdominal wall until the
psoas has been laid completely bare.

A midaxillary subcostal incision is preferred for the insertion of the
balloon for the following reasons: (i) most surgeons are familiar with the
surgical anatomy of this region and the lumbodorsal fascia (which is
particularly tough here) provides a palpable landmark during blunt dissection; (ii) if the retroperitoneoscopic procedure has to be abandoned,
the incision can be conveniently enlarged; and (iii) being centrally placed,
it allows placement of all the ports by a digital guidance technique. It also
allows digital stripping of the parietal peritoneum off the anterior
abdominal wall, which sometimes may be required before placing the
anterior ports [9].

OPENING UP THE SUBFASCIAL PLANE
The retroperitoneal space is inspected for any accidental peritoneal tear
with a fibreoptic light and small deep retractors. The fascia transversalis
or the Gerota's fascia is picked up with haemostats, incised with scissors
and the subfascial plane opened up with Hegar's dilators [10]. Picking up
Gerota's fascia is made easier if the anaesthetist momentarily interrupts
the patient's breathing in full inspiration. In thin and young patients the
fascia transversalis can even be brought out above the skin level (Fig. 2.4).

PLACEMENT OF THE BALLOON
A balloon mounted on a catheter can be easily placed into the subfascial
retroperitoneal space by gentle pushing. Wetting the balloon aids its introduction. A Gaur balloon is inserted by mounting it over a 5-mm suction

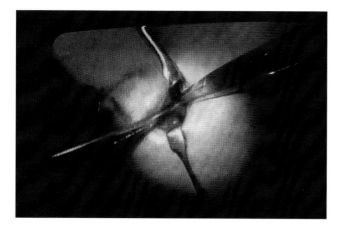

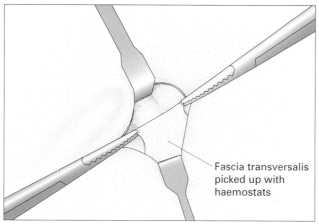

Fascia transversalis
picked up with
haemostats

Fig. 2.4 The fascia transversalis is picked up with haemostats
after retracting the edges with small deep retractors.

irrigation cannula or by gently holding it at its tip with a haemostat and
stretching it. To prevent the balloon from migrating into the extrafascial
space during inflation, the haemostats holding the edges of the fascia are
crossed over the balloon.

EXPANSION AND DISSECTION OF THE RETROPERITONEAL SPACE
The balloon is connected to a sphygmomanometer bulb and is inflated by
squeezing the bulb 15–30 times (Fig. 2.5), depending upon the size of the
patient and the procedure being undertaken. In a patient of average build,
one should not exceed 30 pumpings (about 1000ml), as over-inflation
might tear the peritoneum. It may be difficult to measure the exact
volume with pneumatic inflation; therefore, appreciating the migration of
the balloon down to the anterior superior spine and across to the midline
is a better guide to a safe upper limit. Although we have found pneumatic
inflation of a low-pressure balloon to be safe in our hands, if there is a
particular concern about the theoretical risk of air embolism due to
balloon rupture, the balloon can alternatively be inflated with fluid using
a 50-ml syringe.

The balloon is left inflated for about 5 minutes to allow for haemostasis. Thereafter, it is deflated and removed. If the balloon ruptures

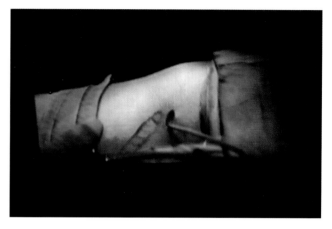

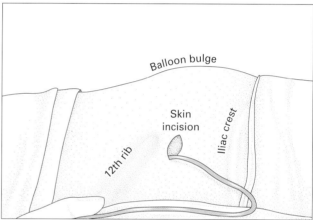

Fig. 2.5 A glove balloon has been inflated with air in the lumbar retroperitoneal space using a sphygmomanometer bulb.

during inflation, a second balloon should be inflated as soon as possible to prevent formation of a film of clotted blood over the tissues.

MONITORING BALLOON INFLATION

Monitoring balloon pressures during inflation is not mandatory, but is advisable during the early part of the learning curve. This is done by connecting the balloon to a manometer through a three-way adapter. However, the clinical monitoring of the patient during balloon inflation is of the utmost significance. The patient's pulse and blood pressure, the amount of bleeding around the side of the balloon, the migration of the balloon and the amount of force required to inflate it are important clinical parameters which should be routinely monitored. In a patient of average build, the balloon is palpable at 200 ml and visible at 300 ml of inflation. It gradually migrates medially and inferiorly like an enlarging spleen and reaches the midline and the level of the anterior superior spine at about 1000 ml. If the balloon is not migrating as expected, or if undue force is being required, it should be deflated to ensure that it has been placed properly. Normally, no more than a few drops of blood come out by the side of the balloon during its inflation, but if there is a continuous ooze it should be left inflated for a longer period to encourage haemostasis.

ESTABLISHMENT OF THE PRIMARY PORT AND PRELIMINARY
RETROPERITONEOSCOPY

If there had been any oozing during balloon inflation, the retroperitoneal
space is mopped out with a small wet gauze on a haemostat, or washed
and sucked out with a sump sucker [11]. A 10- or 12-mm port is then
established by introducing a Hasson-type cannula into the retroperitoneal
space. Alternatively, the incision can be made airtight around an ordinary
cannula with interrupted sutures or with a purse-string suture. The latter
is more useful, as it can be easily undone and redone for intra-operative
dismantling of the primary port, which is sometimes required for
mopping the retroperitoneal space or digital exploration [11].

The primary port is connected to a pneumoinsufflator with the pressure
set at 10–15 mmHg. A preliminary retroperitoneoscopy is performed to
assess the quality of the balloon dissection, detect the presence of a
peritoneal tear or other tissue damage and to locate any debris if the
balloon had burst. The balloon dissection is repeated if it is inadequate.

The appearance at this stage depends on the initial balloon placement.
1 *Extrafascial balloon dissection.* The anatomical landmarks are masked
by the fascia. Only the muscles of the posterior abdominal wall with the
overlying nerves and the iliac artery are seen (Fig. 2.6). If the patient is
slim, the renal silhouette or a ureteral stone bulge can also be made out.

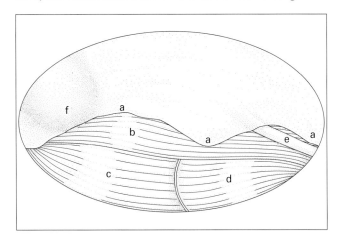

Fig. 2.6 Schematic view of the retroperitoneal space dissected
with the balloon placed extrafascially: **a**, the reflected parietal
peritoneum and the fascia; **b**, psoas; **c**, quadratus lumborum;
d, iliacus; **e**, iliac artery; and **f**, the renal silhouette.

2 *Subfascial balloon dissection.* If the balloon has been placed deep to
Gerota's fascia or fascia transversalis, a variety of retroperitoneal
structures can be exposed by the balloon, depending upon the quality of
the subfascial space created initially and the presence of retroperitoneal
inflammatory adhesions (Figs 2.7 and 2.8). With an optimal dissection,
the adrenal bulge, the whole of the posterior surface of the kidney, the
renal pelvis covered with fat, the entire abdominal ureter, the gonadal
vein, the inferior vena cava and the aorta can be seen. The inferior
mesenteric vessels can sometimes be seen in thin subjects.

The iliac approach

PATIENT POSITION

The anaesthetized patient is placed in a supine position with a sandbag

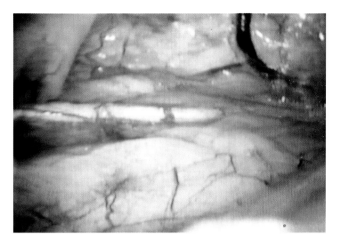

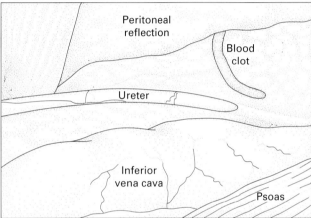

Fig. 2.7 View of the retroperitoneal space dissected with the balloon placed subfascially. The ureter and the inferior vena cava have been neatly dissected by the balloon. The psoas, the reflected parietal peritoneum and a blood clot can also be seen.

under the ipsilateral buttock to provide an approximate 30° tilt to the pelvis.

POSITION OF THE SURGICAL TEAM AND EQUIPMENT
This is identical to the subumbilical lumbar approach.

PORT SITES
A 2-cm oblique incision is made at McBurney's point for insertion of the balloon and the primary port (Fig. 2.9). McBurney's point is selected as it allows digital dissection of the pelvic retroperitoneum almost up to the midline and makes conversion to an open procedure much easier. Incisions for the secondary ports are marked above the iliac crest in the anterior axillary line and in the inguinal region just medial to the anterior superior spine. If required, a third port can be placed in the lumbar region in the midaxillary line (Fig. 2.9).

CREATION OF THE INITIAL RETROPERITONEAL SPACE
The skin incision is deepened by blunt dissection until the external oblique aponeurosis is exposed. This is incised for about 2 cm, its edges separated with a haemostat and retracted with small right-angled retractors. The fibres of internal oblique and transversus abdominis are

separated by blunt dissection with the haemostat until the retroperitoneal space is entered. The index finger is introduced into the retroperitoneal space, which is enlarged by digital dissection of the parietal peritoneum, first laterally and then posteriorly until it has been lifted off the psoas and the pulsations of the iliac artery can be felt. For better exposure of the pelvic retroperitoneum, the digital dissection of the peritoneum is extended medially until the sacral promontory can be felt. If the digital dissection of the peritoneum is carried out anteriorly towards the pubic symphysis, a good exposure of the bladder and a limited exposure of the retropubic space can be obtained.

PLACEMENT OF THE BALLOON

The parietal peritoneum is retracted with a small Deaver retractor and the balloon, mounted on a catheter or a 5-mm blunt instrument, is introduced into the retroperitoneal space anterior to iliopsoas. The remaining steps of the procedure are identical to those used for a lumbar retroperitoneoscopy.

The approach provides an excellent view of iliopsoas, the iliac arteries, the mid ureter, the gonadal vein, the vas deferens and the bladder (Fig. 2.10).

The suprapubic approach

PATIENT POSITION

The anaesthetized and catheterized patient is positioned over the break in the operating table to open up the suprapubic space. A slight Trendelenburg tilt displaces the intestines cranially. The thighs are abducted to provide vaginal access if a bladder neck suspension is planned.

POSITION OF THE SURGICAL TEAM AND EQUIPMENT

This is similar to that for an iliac procedure except that the surgeon and the first assistant stand on the contralateral side for better manoeuvrability.

PORT SITES

A 2-cm transverse skin incision is made in the suprapubic region for insertion of the balloon and the primary port. Marks are made in the infraumbilical and the iliac regions lateral to the inferior epigastric vessels for the three secondary ports (Fig. 2.11(a)).

CREATION OF THE INITIAL RETROPERITONEAL SPACE

The incision is deepened by blunt dissection until the linea alba is exposed. A 2-cm incision is made in the linea alba and the suprapubic space is entered and opened up with a haemostat. The index finger is introduced into the cave of Retzius and the parietal peritoneum stripped off the bladder, the anterior abdominal wall and the pelvis by digital dissection.

PLACEMENT OF THE BALLOON

The balloon is placed into the cave of Retzius. The rest of the procedure is

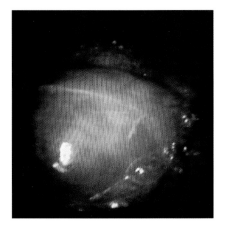

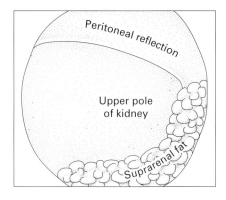

Fig. 2.8 The upper pole of the kidney and the suprarenal fat have been exposed following subfascial balloon dissection.

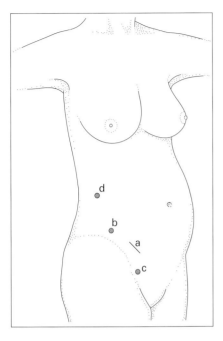

Fig. 2.9 Patient position and port placement for iliac retroperitoneoscopy: **a**, incision for the balloon and the primary port; **b**, the iliac port; **c**, the inguinal port; and **d**, the lumbar port.

identical to the other approaches. The urinary bladder, pubic symphysis and iliac vessels can be easily identified as soon as the laparoscope is introduced (Fig. 2.11(b)).

The closed percutaneous balloon access technique

Suprailiac approach

McDougall and colleagues use a percutaneous access technique to first establish a 12-mm primary port through the inferior lumbar triangle under fluoroscopic control. The retroperitoneal space is then dissected with the tip of the telescope and a balloon, made from the middle finger of a surgical glove loaded inside an Amplatz sheath, is placed into the space. The retroperitoneal space is dissected further by inflating the balloon [12].

Subcostal approach

The author uses the subcostal approach which, like its 'mini open' counterpart, involves neither 'blind' Veress needle or trocar puncture nor

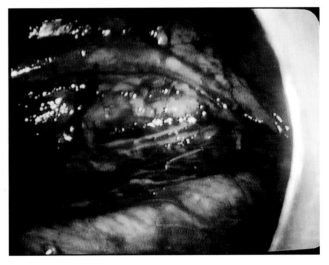

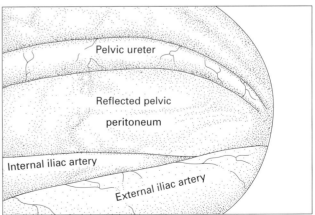

Fig. 2.10 View of the left iliac retroperitoneum following balloon dissection: the pelvic ureter; the external iliac artery; the internal iliac artery; and the reflected pelvic peritoneum.

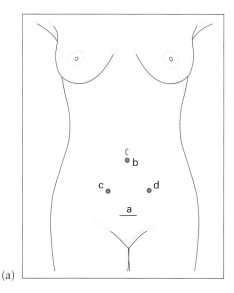

(a)

Fig. 2.11 (a) Patient position and port placement for suprapubic retroperitoneoscopy: **a**, incision for the balloon and the suprapubic port; **b**, the subumbilical port; and **c,d**, the iliac ports. (b) The left retropubic space after balloon dissection: the pubic ramus; the distended bladder; and the reflected peritoneum.

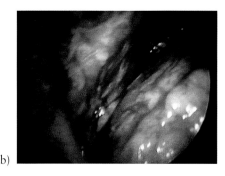

(b)

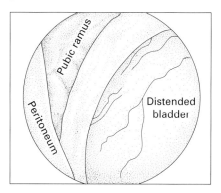

fluoroscopy [13]. A 10-mm subcostal incision is made in the midaxillary plane and the retroperitoneal space is entered with a haemostat, as in the mini open technique. The track is dilated with a blunt obturator or a Hegar's dilator, which is also used to blindly open up the retroperitoneal space over the anterior surface of psoas. A 10-mm blunt port is then pushed through the track into the retroperitoneal space. Pneumoinsufflation is started at 20mmHg pressure and the retroperitoneal space is further dissected towards the target in the subfascial plane with the tip of the telescope (Fig. 2.12). The balloon is inserted through the cannula, which is then removed to allow unrestricted expansion of the balloon.

Although percutaneous access provides a leak-proof primary port with better cosmetic results, subfascial placement of the balloon is often not possible. A further disadvantage of this technique is that it does not permit digital exploration of the space.

Variants of the balloon technique

The condom dissection technique

The author uses this technique to perform balloon dissection of the retroperitoneal space under vision [14]. The balloon is slipped over the distal end

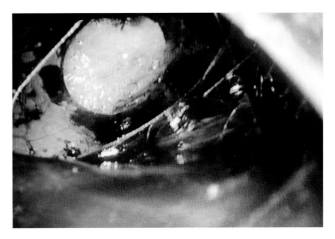

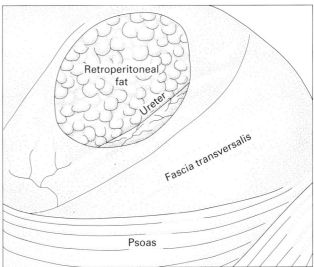

Fig. 2.12 View of the left lumbar retroperitoneum following a blind percutaneous blunt dissection: psoas and the fascia transversalis with a hole created during the blind dissection. The retroperitoneal fat and the ureter can be seen through the hole.

of a 10-mm laparoscopic cannula by slightly stretching it, like a condom. The assembly is introduced into the retroperitoneal space by the mini open technique. A 10-mm laparoscope is introduced into the cannula up to its tip and the balloon is then inflated with air using a sphygmomanometer bulb. Continuous laparoscopic monitoring of the retroperitoneal balloon dissection is possible with this technique. A limited blunt dissection of the retroperitoneal space can also be carried out through the balloon using the tip of the telescope or a blunt dissector introduced through the working channel of an angled telescope.

We do not routinely use the technique as it adds to the operating time without any significant advantage. The dissection from inside the balloon is not very effective and if the balloon has not been placed in the right plane at the first instance, it may not be easy to correctly reinsert the assembly.

Selective balloon dissection

Primary selective balloon dissection is performed by inflating the balloon after placing it over the target area. The expanding balloon can be selectively made to migrate to the lower or the upper abdomen by manually obliterating the upper or the lower retroperitoneal space, respectively [5].

Secondary selective balloon dissection may be performed if the primary dissection is unsatisfactory. This can be done by inflating a double balloon [15] or by inflating the balloon placed over the target area after manually obliterating the already dissected retroperitoneal space. However, it should be appreciated that both methods force the balloon to expand in a restricted space and could thereby cause tissue damage.

The balloon access technique simplifies retroperitoneal laparoscopy by creating a retroperitoneal space and neatly dissecting the retroperitoneal structures at the same time. It is safe provided the balloon is inflated in a virgin retroperitoneal space. However, peritoneal or vascular damage might occur if the balloon is not allowed to expand freely due to retroperitoneal adhesions or is forced to expand in a particular direction by obliteration of part of the space by manual compression or inflating a second balloon.

References

1 Gaur DD. Laparoscopic operative retroperitoneoscopy: Use of a new device. *J Urol* 1992; 148: 1137–1139.

2 Wickham JEA. The surgical treatment of renal lithiasis. In: Wickham JEA, ed. *Urinary Calculus Disease*. New York: Churchill Livingstone, 1979: 145–198.

3 Clayman RV, Kavoussi LR, Soper NJ, Albala DM, Figenshau RS, Chandhoke PS. Laparoscopic nephrectomy: Review of the initial 10 cases. *J Endourol* 1992; 6: 127–131.

4 Mandressi A, Buizza C, Zaroli A, Bernasconi S, Antonelli D, Bellni M. Laparoscopic nephrectomies and adrenalectomies by posterior retro-extra-peritoneal approach. *J Endourol* 1993; 7 (supplement): S174.

5 Gaur DD. Retroperitoneoscopy: the balloon technique. *Ann R Coll Surg Engl* 1994; 76: 259–263.

6 Gaur DD, Agarwal DK, Kulkarni SB, Purohit KC, Shah HK. Retroperitoneoscopy: The dynamics of balloon dissection. Presentation at BAUS annual meeting, Birmingham, July 1994.

7 Eden CG. Operative retroperitoneoscopy. *Br J Urol* 1995; 76: 125–130.

8 Gaur DD, Agarwal DK, Purohit KC. Retroperitoneal laparoscopic nephrectomy: Initial case report. *J Urol* 1993; 149: 103–105.

9 Gaur DD, Agarwal DK, Purohit KC, Darshane AS. Retroperitoneal laparoscopic pyelolithotomy. *J Urol* 1994; 154: 927–929.

10 Gaur DD. The use of Hegar's dilators in laparoscopy. *Min Invas Ther* 1993; 2: 333–334.

11 Gaur DD. Retroperitoneal laparoscopy: some technical modifications. *Br J Urol* 1996; 77: 304–306.

12 McDougall EM, Clayman RV, Fadden PT. Retroperitoneoscopy: The Washington University Medical School experience. *Urology* 1994; 43: 446–452.

13 Gaur DD. Retroperitoneal laparoscopy: a simple technique of balloon insertion and establishment of the primary port (unpublished observations).

14 Gaur DD, Agarwal DK, Purohit KC. Laparoscopic condom dissection: a new technique of retroperitoneoscopy. *J Endourol* 1994; 8: 149–151.

15 Gill IS, Munch LC, Lucas BA, Das S. Retroperitoneoscopic nephroureterectomy: the double balloon technique. *J Endourol* 1994; 6 (supplement): 161.

3 Anaesthesia

B. M. P. RADEMAKER

Until recently, laparoscopy was performed in healthy young women undergoing diagnostic or minor therapeutic gynaecological procedures, presenting few challenges in anaesthetic management. The development of new laparoscopic techniques, such as extraperitoneal laparoscopy, which involve lengthy procedures not only in healthy young patients but also in the elderly, has prompted an interest in the pathophysiological effects of these procedures. In this chapter these effects and their impact on anaesthetic management are discussed.

Pathophysiological effects

Haemodynamics

Haemodynamics are affected during transperitoneal laparoscopy by the creation of a pneumoperitoneum. Both the mechanical (pressure) and pharmacological effects of the insufflated gas are important. Initially, pneumoperitoneum will 'squeeze' venous blood in the abdomen back to the heart. Thereafter the increase in intra-abdominal pressure results in reduced blood flow in the inferior vena cava and pooling of blood in the legs. The composite of both of these mechanical effects on venous return causes an increase followed by a decrease in cardiac output. Compression of the aorta and the large intestinal arteries results in an increase in systemic vascular resistance (SVR) and a reduction of cardiac output [1]. In addition to the mechanical effects, absorption of the insufflated gas will pharmacologically affect haemodynamics [2]. Sympathetic stimulation secondary to increased levels of arterial carbon dioxide (CO_2) following absorption from the peritoneal cavity causes increases in arterial blood pressure and SVR.

There are no data on the effects of extraperitoneal laparoscopy on haemodynamics. Preliminary data of an experimental study in pigs showed significant differences between extraperitoneal laparoscopy and its conventional transperitoneal counterpart. In contrast to the use of a conventional pneumoperitoneum, the extraperitoneal instillation of CO_2 to maintain an extraperitoneal cavity was associated with smaller increases in central filling pressures (Fig.3.1). Cardiac output and heart rate were affected equally by the conventional and extraperitoneal approaches. These

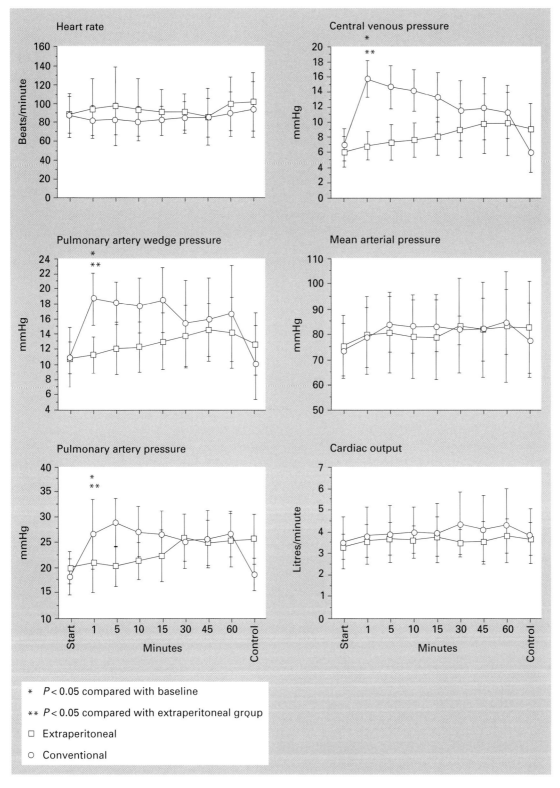

Fig. 3.1 Haemodynamic parameters during 60-minute CO_2 insufflation at 14 mmHg in pigs, either extra- ($n = 8$) or intraperitoneal ($n = 8$), demonstrating that extraperitoneal insufflation is associated with significantly lower filling pressures.

findings suggest that the extraperitoneal approach might result in less cardiovascular impairment than conventional laparoscopy.

Patient position and several additional factors, such as mode of ventilation, choice of anaesthetic agents and adequacy of intravascular volume, may modify the haemodynamic responses to pneumoperitoneum [1]. Upper abdominal laparoscopic surgery is usually performed in the reverse Trendelenburg ('head-up') position, which causes a decrease in cardiac output [1]. Extraperitoneal laparoscopy may be easier to perform in the prone position. In an experimental study in pigs performed to investigate the haemodynamic effects of the prone position during CO_2 pneumoperitoneum, the author found that laparoscopy in the prone position caused no greater haemodynamic depression than its supine counterpart [3].

Cardiac dysrhythmia

Hypercarbia secondary to the absorption of CO_2 may provoke cardiac dysrhythmias. Although extraperitoneal laparoscopy tends to result in greater CO_2 absorption, and the tendency toward hypercarbia is thus greater, no adverse clinical effects have been reported.

Pulmonary mechanics

Transperitoneal laparoscopy affects pulmonary mechanics and gas exchange both during the procedure and in the post-operative period. The cephalad movement of the diaphragm during pneumoperitoneum results in a reduction of lung compliance. In addition, the 'head-down' position decreases functional residual capacity and total lung volume. Theoretically, the prone position might also impede movement of the diaphragm. We observed no differences in lung compliance using either the prone or the supine position [3].

Laparoscopic surgery is associated with less compromise of post-operative lung function as compared with open surgery. In the context of cholecystectomy, the adoption of a laparoscopic approach leads to a reduction of impairment of post-operative lung function of 30–40% [4,5]. Data on lung function following extraperitoneal laparoscopy are not yet available. The mechanisms of lung dysfunction after surgery appear to be multifactorial. Possible causes of better lung performance after laparoscopic surgery are improved diaphragmatic function, smaller wounds and reduced pain.

Gas exchange, hypoxia and respiratory acidosis

Hypoxia may occur during laparoscopy because of increased ventilation/perfusion mismatching and intrapulmonary shunting. However, the incidence of clinically significant hypoxia during laparoscopy is low. In contrast, increased arterial $P\text{CO}_2$ ($Pa\text{CO}_2$) with respiratory acidosis has frequently been reported during CO_2 pneumoperitoneum. In healthy patients undergoing laparoscopic cholecystectomy, minute ventilation had to be increased by 12–16% in order to maintain Pa_{CO_2} close to pre-insufflation levels. Patients with cardiopulmonary disease are more likely to develop hypercarbia. Extraperitoneal CO_2 insufflation may result in considerably higher Pa_{CO_2} as compared with conventional pneumoperitoneum [6]. However, an experimental study in dogs did not show higher arterial CO_2 levels during extraperitoneal insufflation compared with conventional pneumoperitoneum. Three mechanisms may contribute to the development of hypercarbia: (i) systemic absorption of CO_2; (ii) increased dead space ventilation; and (iii) the development of subcutaneous emphysema [7].

Metabolic responses

Surgery stimulates a series of hormonal, metabolic and immunological responses that together constitute the stress response. Anaesthesia may attenuate this response to surgery, although its influence is limited compared to the effects of surgery. It is conceivable that reducing the size of the surgical wound may reduce the release of these mediators. Since laparoscopic surgery is associated with smaller incisions, it has been speculated that the metabolic endocrine response can be attenuated by this type of surgery. This might at least partly explain the fact that laparoscopically operated patients resume normal life earlier. Indeed, parts of the acute-phase reaction are attenuated after laparoscopic cholecystectomy as compared with the open procedure [8]. However, the catabolic hormones cortisol, adrenocorticotrophic hormone (ACTH) and adrenaline appear to respond in a similar fashion after open or laparoscopic cholecystectomy [8,9]. Data on the metabolic endocrine response to extraperitoneal laparoscopic surgery are not available.

Post-operative pain

Post-operative pain is decreased following transperitoneal laparoscopic surgery as compared with pain after the open procedure. The reduction of pain in laparoscopically operated patients observed in most studies resulted in an up to fivefold decrease in analgesic consumption. A decreased analgesic requirement has also been reported following an extraperitoneal laparoscopic approach for inguinal hernia repair [10].

Post-operative nausea

Nausea is one of the most frequently observed minor sequelae after transperitoneal laparoscopy, with a reported incidence ranging from 38 to 80%. The incidence of nausea following extraperitoneal laparoscopic surgery has not yet been well defined.

Gas embolism

Fatal complications resulting from laparoscopy are rare [11]. Gas embolism is the most feared complication with a reported incidence of 0.015% in gynaecology [12]. Characteristic signs of gas embolism are a 'mill-wheel' murmur and a decreased end-tidal CO_2 ($EtCO_2$) due to increased dead space ventilation and reduced cardiac output. These events may be followed by cyanosis, dysrhythmias and circulatory collapse. The combination of precordial Doppler ultrasound monitoring with capnography provides the earliest and most sensitive non-invasive method of detecting gas embolism. Early recognition of gas embolism is of paramount importance.

Immediate treatment consists of switching off the CO_2 gas supply and deflating the laparoscopic workspace. Administration of nitrous oxide should be discontinued and hyperventilation of the lungs with 100% oxygen commenced to counteract the effects of the increased dead space and the large amounts of systemically absorbed CO_2. If the circulatory status does not improve immediately the patient should be placed in the left lateral head-down position: Durant's manoeuvre. This position will place the right ventricular outflow tract below the rest of the right ventricle, which may result in terminating the gas lock. However, placing the patient in a left lateral position may be impossible during laparoscopic surgery performed in the prone or lateral positions. The alternative manoeuvre is aspiration of trapped gas via a central venous catheter. As the treatment of a large gas embolism is difficult, the management of this complication should be directed towards the prevention of the problem. Insufflation of gas should not exceed a rate of 1 litre/minute before confirmation of the correct position of the insufflation needle.

Pneumothorax, pneumopericardium, pneumomediastinum and subcutaneous emphysema

Complications affecting the anaesthetic management of the patient were rarely observed during diagnostic laparoscopy. Unilateral and bilateral tension pneumothorax, pneumopericardium, pneumomediastinum and subcutaneous emphysema are now much more frequently encountered, especially following extraperitoneal laparoscopy [13–15]. Pneumothorax, pneumopericardium or tension pneumomediastinum may result in a life-threatening situation, secondary to compression of the heart and great veins. After release of pneumoperitoneum or pneumoretroperitoneum, subcutaneous emphysema, mediastinal emphysema and pneumopericardium are generally self-limiting and require no therapeutic intervention. Post-operatively, patients may complain of substernal chest pain, cervical pain, back pain or dyspnoea. Prolonged mechanical ventilation is necessary when massive subcutaneous emphysema is present, causing ventilatory impairment.

Anaesthetic management

Planning and pre-operative evaluation

Evaluation and optimization of pre-existing cardiovascular disease is mandatory since laparoscopy causes haemodynamic changes which might precipitate a latent cardiovascular crisis. The choice of whether to use an open or laparoscopic approach in patients with severe cardiac disease must be made after weighing the adverse effects of laparoscopic insufflation against the post-operative benefits of early mobilization. In patients with chronic pulmonary disease, laparoscopic surgery is the treatment of choice because of the lesser impairment of lung function. During the laparoscopic procedure these patients may develop hypercarbia or hypoxia. However, these disadvantages are outweighed by the positive effects of laparoscopic surgery on post-operative lung function.

Anaesthetic technique

General anaesthesia is advocated in patients undergoing laparoscopic surgery. Intubation of the trachea with mechanical ventilation is routinely performed in these patients. The use of a laryngeal mask with mechanical ventilation cannot be advocated for two reasons: (i) displacement of the mask may allow the stomach to distend with CO_2 making upper abdominal laparoscopic surgery difficult; and (ii) the laryngeal mask should not be used when the patient is prone or during procedures exceeding 30 minutes because of the risk of passive regurgitation. Patients undergoing laparoscopy are at risk of aspiration of stomach contents because of the increased intra-abdominal pressure during the procedure. During gynaecological laparoscopy regurgitation of quantities of stomach contents large enough to produce aspiration pneumonia has been demonstrated. However, there are no reports of an increased incidence of aspiration pneumonia after laparoscopy.

REGIONAL ANAESTHESIA
Although epidural anaesthesia has been successfully used during gynaecological laparoscopy, four of the seven patients reported shoulder pain [16]. Another study has reported the successful use of epidural anaesthesia for laparoscopic cholecystectomy in patients with cystic fibrosis [17]. The combination of thoracic epidural analgesia with general anaesthesia was not associated with a beneficial effect on post-operative lung function, although post-operative pain control was better than with intramuscular opioids [4]. The difficulty of blocking shoulder pain with regional anaesthesia and the inability to control ventilation limits its application as a sole anaesthetic modality during laparoscopic surgery.

Choice of anaesthetic agent

The ideal anaesthetic technique for laparoscopy would result in high patient acceptance, avoidance of the pain of injection, no awareness during surgery, no nausea and vomiting, good post-operative analgesia and an early recovery. In addition, haemodynamics would not be affected. Lung function would be preserved and the catabolic state diminished or even abolished by attenuating the metabolic endocrine response. The anaesthetic technique should be safe when used in combination with CO_2 insufflation. Although no single anaesthetic agent emerges from the literature as being the perfect choice, it appears that propofol is associated with rapid recovery and reduces the incidence of post-operative side-effects, such as nausea and vomiting.

It has been suggested that it might be advantageous to use an anaesthetic agent which causes mild vasodilatation, without depressing the myocardium. This might at least partly counteract the adverse effects of the haemodynamic changes associated with CO_2 pneumoperitoneum. Both isoflurane and propofol possess these properties. No study comparing these two agents for laparoscopy has yet been conducted but isoflurane has the least myocardial depressant properties of the commonly used inhalational anaesthetic agents. Halothane anaesthesia may potentiate the adverse haemodynamic effects of pneumoperitoneum and may also sensitize the heart to dysrhythmias. Its use during laparoscopy is therefore best avoided.

No single anaesthetic technique can prevent the impairment of pulmonary function after abdominal surgery. Neither is any anaesthetic agent capable of effectively attenuating the metabolic endocrine response to surgical stress. However, the α_2-adrenoreceptor agonist dexmedetomidine has recently been shown to decrease the metabolic endocrine response to gynaecological laparoscopy.

The use of nitrous oxide (N_2O) as part of the *anaesthetic* technique for laparoscopy is controversial. Its use has been associated with an increased frequency of post-operative nausea, although this has not been confirmed in a large survey [18]. Furthermore, N_2O is known to accumulate in cavities, which may result in dilatation of the bowel. In theory, this might obscure vision during prolonged laparoscopy, although it was recently demonstrated that this is not the case [19]. Of greater concern is the report of an intra-abdominal explosion occurring during a laparoscopic procedure in which the pneumoperitoneum was created using N_2O [20]. In addition, it has been shown that when N_2O is used as part of the anaesthetic regimen during laparoscopy sufficient concentrations of N_2O are reached intra-abdominally to support combustion. Consequently, N_2O should not be used during laparoscopic procedures that might require electrocoagulation.

Vasoactive drugs

Early treatment of hypotension during laparoscopy should consist of desufflation of the pneumoperitoneum and placing the patient in a head-down position to increase venous return. Vasoactive drugs which possess both α- and β-adrenergic agonist activity, such as ephedrine and metaraminol, are helpful in the treatment of sudden hypotensive periods. As hypovolaemia is known to aggravate markedly the adverse effects of pneumoperitoneum, fluid resuscitation is necessary to correct hypo-volaemia when hypotension occurs.

Prolonged haemodynamic instability, especially in patients with under-lying cardiovascular disease, may require the administration of vasoactive drugs for a longer period. In theory, dobutamine should be the first choice for treating a low cardiac output state with normal to high arterial pressure during laparoscopy. Its β-agonist activity causes both increased cardiac contractility and decreased SVR. Dopamine should be the first choice in a patient with a low cardiac output and low arterial blood pressure.

Nitroglycerine and nitroprusside may also be used to reduce afterload, which is achieved through a direct effect on vascular smooth muscle. However, the use of vasodilators may reduce preload, causing a further decrease in cardiac output and decreased SVR, which might result in hypotension. There are no data on the effects of different vasoactive agents during laparoscopic surgery. Vasoactive drugs, especially vasodilators, should be used with caution during laparoscopic surgery.

Monitoring

During every laparoscopic procedure standard monitoring should consist of an electrocardiogram, non-invasive blood pressure measurement, pulse oximetry and continuous measurement of $EtCO_2$ by capnography, to provide a basis for adjustments to ventilation. Although capnography effectively measures $EtCO_2$ levels, there may be a considerable under-estimation of arterial CO_2. This indicates that $EtCO_2$ values should be interpreted with caution.

During extraperitoneal laparoscopy frequent blood-gas analysis is necessary in most patients, and especially those with underlying cardio-pulmonary disease. Insertion of an arterial catheter to obtain serial blood samples is indicated under these circumstances; this also allows for continuous blood pressure monitoring. Advanced haemodynamic mon-itoring using a pulmonary artery catheter to allow cardiac output and SVR to be calculated is recommended in patients with severe cardiac disease. At our institution, a central venous catheter is inserted in every patient undergoing laparoscopy in the prone position, to allow possible CO_2 emboli to be treated. It should be appreciated that the central venous pressure during laparoscopy is raised. It does not reflect the true intra-vascular volume status and pressure values may therefore be misleading.

Post-operative monitoring

Ideally, in the post-operative period patients should be observed closely for a period at least as long as the surgical procedure. Heart rate, blood pressure, respiration rate and arterial oxygen saturation should be measured. In patients who show signs of subcutaneous gas (crepitus) a chest X-ray should be obtained to investigate the possibility of mediastinal emphysema, pneumopericardium or pneumothorax. If one of these is present, prolonged observation of the patient and blood-gas analysis is indicated. Usually these sequelae resolve without treatment and no specific interventions are necessary. In the presence of extensive emphysema that might compromise ventilation, prolonged intubation with assisted ventilation is necessary.

References

1 Joris JL, Noirot DP, Legrand MJ, Jacquet NJ, Lamy ML. Haemodynamic changes during laparoscopic cholecystectomy. *Anesth Analg* 1993; 76: 1067–1071.

2 Rademaker BMP, Odoom JA, de Wit L, Kalkman CJ, ten Brinks S, Ringers J. Haemodynamic effects of pneumoperitoneum for laparoscopic surgery: a comparison of CO_2 with N_2O insufflation. *Eur J Anaesthesiol* 1994; 11: 301–306.

3 Bannenberg JJG, Rademaker BMP, Grundeman PF, Kalkman CJ, Meijer DW, Klopper PJ. Hemodynamics during laparoscopy in the supine or prone position. An experimental study. *Surg Endosc* 1995; 9: 125–127.

4 Rademaker BMP, Ringers J, Odoom JA, de Wit L, Kalkman CJ, Oosting J. Pulmonary function and stress response after laparoscopic cholecystectomy: comparison with subcostal incision and influence of thoracic epidural analgesia. *Anesth Analg* 1992; 75: 381–385.

5 Schauer PR, Luna J, Ghiatas AA, Glen ME, Warren JM, Sirinek KR. Pulmonary function after laparoscopic cholecystectomy. *Surgery* 1993; 114: 389–397.

6 Mullett CE, Viale JP, Sagnard PE. Pulmonary CO_2 elimination during surgical procedures using intra- or extraperitoneal CO_2 insufflation. *Anesth Analg* 1993; 76: 622–626.

7 Lister DV, Rudston-Brown B, Wriner B, McEwen J, Chan M, Whalley K. Carbon dioxide absorption is not linearly related to intraperitoneal carbon dioxide insufflation pressure in pigs. *Anesthesiology* 1994; 80: 129–136.

8 Joris J, Cigarini I, Legrand MJ. Metabolic and respiratory changes after cholecystectomy performed via laparotomy or laparoscopy. *Br J Anaesth* 1992; 69: 341–345.

9 Jakeways MSR, Mitchell V, Hashim IA, Chadwick SJD, Shenkin A. Metabolic and inflammatory responses after open or laparoscopic cholecystectomy. *Br J Surg* 1993; 81: 127–131.

10 Stoker DL, Spiegelhalter DJ, Singh R, Wellwood JM. Laparoscopic versus open inguinal hernia repair: randomised prospective trial. *Lancet* 1994; 343: 1243–1245.

11 Lantz PE, Smith JD. Fatal carbon dioxide embolism complicating attempted laparoscopic cholecystectomy—case report and literature review. *J Forensic Sci* 1994; 39: 1468–1480.

12 Chamberlain GVP, Carren Brown JAC. *Gynaecological Laparoscopy. The Report of the Working Party of the Confidential Enquiry into Gynaecological Laparoscopy*. London: The Royal College of Obstetricians and Gynaecologists of England, 1978.

13 Welter HF, Redling F, Greiner H. Subcutaneous CO_2 emphysema after laparoscopic cholecystectomy. *Der Chirurg* 1993; 64: 209.

14 Woolner DF, Johnson DM. Bilateral pneumothorax and surgical emphysema associated with laparoscopic cholecystectomy. *Anaesth Intensive Care* 1993; 21: 108–110.

15 Noguchi J, Takagi H, Konishi M. Severe subcutaneous emphysema and hypercapnia during laparoscopic cholecystectomy. *Masui* 1993; 42: 602–605.

16 Brampton WJ, Watson RJ. Arterial to end tidal carbon dioxide tension difference during laparoscopy. Magnitude and effects of anaesthetic technique. *Anaesthesia* 1990; 45: 453–456.

17 Edelman DS. Laparoscopic cholecystectomy under continuous epidural anesthesia in patients with cystic fibrosis. *Am J Dis Child* 1991; 145: 723–724.

18 Hovorka J, Korttila K. Nitrous oxide does not increase nausea and vomiting following gynaecological laparoscopy. *Can J Anaesth* 1989; 36: 145–148.

19 Taylor E, Feinstein R, White PF, Soper N. Anaesthesia for laparoscopic cholecystectomy. Is nitrous oxide contraindicated? *Anesthesiology* 1992; 76: 541–543.

20 El-Kady AA, Abd-El-Razek M. Intraperitoneal explosion during female sterilization by laparoscopic electrocoagulation. *Int J Gynaecol* 1976; 14: 487–488.

4

Pelvic lymphadenectomy

T. A. ABDEL-MEGUID & L. G. GOMELLA

Laparoscopic surgery offers the prospect of reduced morbidity and shorter hospital stay. Since it was originally adapted from gynaecological and general surgery, the majority of procedures have been described based on the transperitoneal approach. Early urological laparoscopic procedures, such as pelvic lymph node dissection, bladder neck suspension and nephrectomy [1], have approached the target organs through the peritoneum, in contrast to open urological surgery, which is confined mostly to the extraperitoneal space. While early reports have supported the use of laparoscopic techniques for a variety of procedures, significant potential complications such as bowel or vascular injuries exist when utilizing the transperitoneal approach [2].

Historically, standard staging pelvic lymph node dissection via an open low midline extraperitoneal approach has been shown to have advantages over the open transperitoneal approach. Freiha and Salzman [3] compared open surgical extraperitoneal lymphadenectomy to the intraperitoneal open surgical approach, and they concluded that the extraperitoneal lymphadenectomy was tolerated better, associated with less morbidity, and had fewer immediate post-operative complications. However, the classic open extraperitoneal approach warrants an average hospital stay of 6.8 days, as well as involving substantial risks such as blood transfusion, thromboembolic accidents, wound infection and lymphocoele formation [4,5]. Marshall and associates have popularized the 'mini-laparotomy' approach through a much smaller incision. Although the complications and hospital stay are reduced dramatically, patients still require 48–72 hours in hospital [6].

Multiple studies have addressed the issue of accuracy and outcome of laparoscopic pelvic lymph node dissection (LPLND) when compared to standard open techniques. Lymph node counts have been shown to be similar between the two techniques, with typically an average total of 10 for LPLND [7].

A recent prospective multicentre study [8] assessing the outcome of urological laparoscopic surgery has demonstrated a continued improvement in outcome and a decreased complication rate. The study included three groups of patients, totalling 482, who underwent a variety of laparoscopic urological procedures in three successive phases. The initial experience phase was before 1991 (P1); the second phase was from 1991 to 1992 (P2); and the latest phase was from 1993 to 1994 (P3). LPLND was the most frequently performed procedure. For all procedures (including LPLND), there was an obvious improvement of outcome and decrease in complication rates (Table 4.1). As shown in this and similar laparoscopic outcome studies, many of the complications are related to the transperitoneal approach. Attempts have been made to utilize the extraperitoneal route, in an effort to further improve the outcome and minimize the incidence of complications.

Table 4.1 Outcome of laparoscopic pelvic lymphadenectomy.

	P1	P2	P3
Total cases	105	132	245
Intraperitoneal CO_2	105 (100%)	132 (100%)	212 (86.5%)
Extraperitoneal CO_2	0	0	33 (13.5%)
Node count	10.8 (2–7)	9.4 (2–16)	13 (2–41)
Positive nodes	8.6%	11.5%	13%
OR time (minutes)	162.8 (60–360)	125 (35–355)	91.4 (40–280)
Hospital stay (hours)	45.6 (23–240)	39.3 (23–240)	36.4 (10–120)
Stay <24 hours	23 (22%)	74 (56%)	230 (90.4%)

The earliest instances of extraperitoneal laparoscopic procedures were limited due to inadequate distension of the extraperitoneal space. Techniques to allow endoscopic extraperitoneal dissection of pelvic lymph nodes were first attempted in the 1970s. Hald and Rasmussen [9] were among the first to report this approach for patients with prostate and bladder cancer. However, their procedure was limited to sampling only palpable nodes due to difficulties of visualization and lack of adequate instrumentation and consequently, in many cases, an insufficient specimen was obtained. More recently, Ferzli and associates [10–12] have investigated the extraperitoneal laparoscopic approach for staging pelvic lymphadenectomy. This group uses blunt entry into the preperitoneal space (Hasson technique) [13], insufflation to 8mmHg, and creation of a space by a combination of blunt and sharp dissection using an operating laparoscope. Due to frequent cleaning to remove blood and debris, this method appears to be more time-consuming and tedious than preliminary distension with a balloon device, described below and in Chapter 2. In addition, the operating laparoscope often can interfere with a portion of the operator's visual field [14]. Moreover, the insufflated gas tends to track along the fascial planes instead of developing the potential space, and inadequate exposure is often a problem.

Gaur [15] was an early advocate of preliminary balloon distension of the extraperitoneal space, utilizing for dissection a cut glove finger mounted on a red rubber catheter. As the peritoneum is attached to the body wall by both delicate and dense fibrous bands, these bands interfere with the ability of simple insufflation to create this potential space. The technique described by Gaur overcomes this obstacle by disrupting these bands. It is this contribution that has led to an expansion in the extraperitoneal laparoscopic approach.

Many manufacturers have developed different styles of trocar-balloon to create the extraperitoneal working space. Our preference is to use the commercially available preperitoneal distension balloon (PDB) (Origin Medsystems, Menlo Park, California, USA) to create this space. The PDB (see Fig. 1.4) consists of a blunt 10 mm extended length laparoscopic trocar with a balloon mounted at its distal end. The initial balloon design was latex rubber, while the latest version is made of silicone, which is completely transparent and more durable. The balloon can be gradually inflated to a volume of 700–1000 ml via a side port with the supplied manual inflation bulb. The design of the PDB trocar allows the insertion of the laparoscope through the shaft of the trocar; and the clear balloon allows laparoscopic visualization and position control while the distension is underway. Other workers have used devices, such as a Foley catheter balloon [16] or Helmstein balloon catheter [17] to develop the extraperitoneal space. Using the former device, the size of the dissected area is limited by the size of the Foley catheter balloon but both devices lack the advantage of visually controlled distension.

Indications for pelvic lymphadenectomy

Not all patients with localized prostate cancer require a staging lymphadenectomy. The procedure should be reserved for those who are at risk of nodal metastasis and in whom the diagnosis of nodal involvement would alter the proposed treatment, such as radiation therapy or perineal prostatectomy. The following patients would appear to benefit from staging LPLND before initiating one of these therapies [18]: patients with apparently localized disease; prostate specific antigen level > 20 ng/ml; elevated prostatic acid phosphatase level; Gleason score of > 7; enlarged nodes on pelvic imaging studies; and clinical stage C disease. Several centres now use the laparoscopic lymphadenectomy at the same time as the perineal prostatectomy or radioactive seed implantation. Laparoscopic lymphadenectomy appears to have little role if a standard retropubic prostatectomy is planned. Patients with bladder cancer can also be staged by this technique.

We consider that patients who have had prior major open pelvic surgery are not suitable candidates for extraperitoneal laparoscopic node dissection (EPLND). Caution is needed in the EPLND approach in patients with a history of hernia repair or ruptured appendix, since the space may be difficult or impossible to develop. These patients can usually be treated with a transperitoneal laparoscopic approach.

Pre-operative preparation

Informed consent by means of a thorough discussion of the risks, benefits, alternatives and potential complications of laparoscopy and the possibility of open surgery is the initial step in preparing the patient for this and any other laparoscopic intervention. All patients are clearly informed that these procedures are in their earliest stages of development and that the clearly defined indications for these procedures await the results of further studies.

The patients are advised to discontinue aspirin and all other platelet-affecting medications at least 5–7 days prior to surgery. Blood is usually not requested but a type and screen is performed.

Patients are instructed to avoid dairy products and other gas-producing foods for two days before the procedure in order to diminish intestinal distension, and to initiate a clear liquid diet the day prior to admission. Routine bowel preparation with milk of magnesia the day prior to surgery, and enemas on the day of surgery, are usually helpful in decompressing the lower intestine. If immediate perineal prostatectomy is planned should the nodes come back negative on frozen pathological examination, a full bowel preparation is administered the night prior to surgery. All patients receive one dose of a broad-spectrum parenteral antibiotic one hour prior to, and two doses after, the procedure.

Technique of extraperitoneal laparoscopic lymphadenectomy

The patient is placed in the supine position on the operating table and pneumatic leg compression stockings are fitted. General endotracheal anaesthesia is induced and a nasogastric tube and urethral catheter are inserted. After appropriate venous access, the arms are positioned at the patient's side. Care should be taken to properly secure the patient to the table and appropriately pad all pressure areas. The entire abdomen and penoscrotal areas are prepared and draped in a fashion that allows for immediate laparotomy in case of emergency.

A vertical skin incision is made 1–2 cm below the inferior umbilical crease in order to avoid the confluence of the anterior and posterior rectus sheaths at the umbilicus. A vertical incision is preferable in case a laparotomy needs to be performed. The skin incision should be large enough to accommodate a 10/11-mm trocar sheath. The tissues are spread with a Kelly clamp down to the anterior rectus sheath. Two 0 Dexon or Vicryl stay sutures are placed in the anterior rectus sheath on each side of the midline to facilitate retraction and closure upon completion of the procedure. Next, the anterior rectus sheath is incised vertically along the linea alba between the two sutures. The two bellies of the recti are separated by blunt dissection and the index finger is passed behind the recti but anterior to the posterior rectus sheath. Blunt finger dissection is used to create the space between the recti and the posterior sheath.

Although we utilize the PDB, any other balloon type dissecting device can be used. The PDB is lubricated with sterile jelly and passed carefully behind the recti in the space created between the recti and their posterior sheath to enter the preperitoneal space at the level of the arcuate line (Fig. 4.1). We believe that this approach provides a more reliable means of not violating the peritoneal membrane. The peritoneum is densely attached at the level of the umbilicus, making inadvertent entry more likely if an attempt to enter the preperitoneal space is made at the

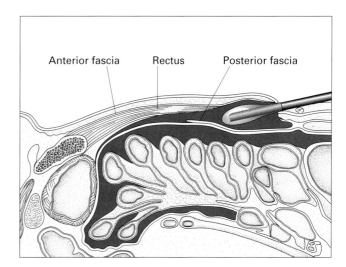

Fig. 4.1 The preperitoneal distension balloon (PDB) enters the preperitoneal space at the level of the arcuate line.

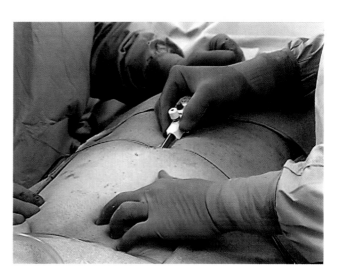

Fig. 4.2 The balloon can be passed inferiorly with external manual guidance down to the pubis. The two holding sutures on the external fascia can be seen.

umbilicus. The balloon can be passed inferiorly with external manual guidance down to the pubis and positioned approximately 2 cm from the pubis (Fig. 4.2).

The balloon is gradually inflated to approximately 700–1000 ml with room air using a manual inflation bulb with the laparoscope in place (Fig. 4.3). An advantage of the PDB system is that the laparoscope-camera unit is inserted through the PDB trocar shaft inside the balloon cavity to visually inspect progress and to ensure adequate dissection and expansion of the space. The distal border of inflation is the pubis and the proximal border is the arcuate line, which is approximately two-thirds of the distance from pubis to umbilicus. The balloon is left inflated for about five minutes to allow for haemostasis, then deflated and the trocar removed. The inflation can be repeated if needed. Occasionally, moving the balloon into the right or left side of the pelvis and inflating in this position can yield more complete lateral dissection.

A 10-mm Hasson-style, blunt-tip trocar (BTT) (Origin Medsystems,

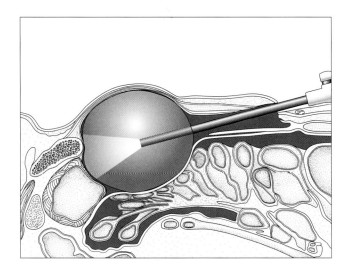

Fig. 4.3 The balloon is gradually inflated to approximately 700–1000 ml with room air using a manual inflation bulb. The laparoscope is held inside the balloon during the inflation to observe for adequate dissection of the space.

Menlo Park, California, USA) is placed in the developed extraperitoneal space. This trocar (Fig. 4.4) has a fascial retention balloon near its distal end and an adjustable sliding foam collar over the shaft. The balloon is inflated with 15–20 ml of room air and, while maintaining outward traction on the inflated balloon against the anterior abdominal wall, the foam collar is pushed forward to lodge in the incision and then locked. The balloon and foam collar work together to seal the incision and effectively prevent leakage of insufflated gas out of the extraperitoneal space (Fig. 4.5). The carbon dioxide (CO_2) insufflator is connected and set to high flow and 8–10 mmHg pressure, which is maintained throughout the procedure. We have recently modified our technique and incorporated the Origin structural Hasson balloon trocar (Fig. 4.6). The design incorporates a structural balloon that provides excellent posterior retraction of the peritoneal contents.

The laparoscope and video system are white-balanced and the end of the lens is coated with an anti-fog solution. The laparoscope is inserted and the preperitoneal space inspected. This usually confirms adequate

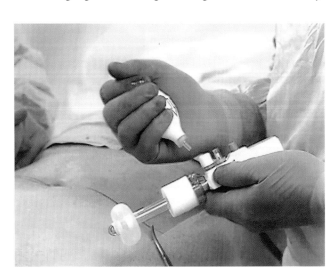

Fig. 4.4 The blunt-tip trocar (BTT) (Origin Medsystems Inc., Menlo Park, California, USA). The fascial retention balloon is inflated with two squeezes of the inflation bulb. The foam collar seals the site at the skin level.

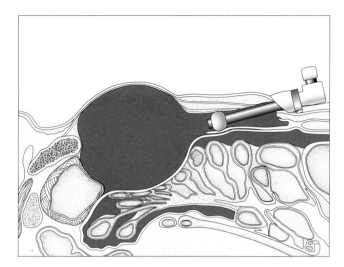

Fig. 4.5 Insufflation through the blunt-tipped Hasson-style trocar maintains the extraperitoneal space.

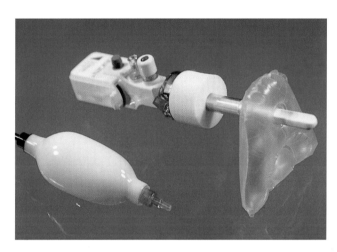

Fig. 4.6 The new Origin structural balloon functions as a Hasson-style cannula. The enlarged fascial retention balloon provides excellent posterior retraction of the peritoneal envelope, facilitating all extraperitoneal laparoscopic procedures.

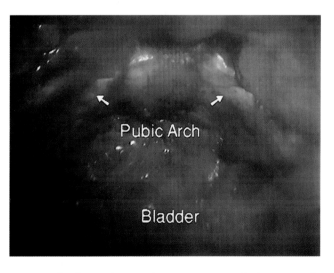

Fig. 4.7 The extraperitoneal space after balloon dissection. The pubic arch is typically seen anteriorly and the bladder posteriorly.

dissection of the space with the pubic arch (Fig. 4.7) and iliac vessels (Fig. 4.8) well visualized. Bleeding is usually minimal and the right side typically dissects more completely than the left. However, a small amount

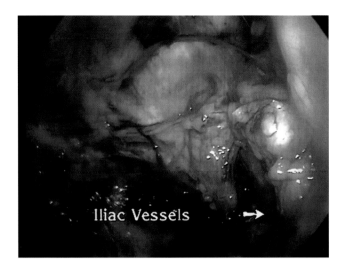

Fig. 4.8 The iliac vessels are seen in the right lower quadrant after balloon dissection.

of blunt dissection may be needed to expose the vessels on the left side.

The pressure is briefly increased to 15 mmHg to facilitate secondary trocar placement, but care should be taken as prolonged pressure at this level may cause tracking of the gas into the subcutaneous tissues. A diamond configuration similar to transperitoneal lymphadenectomy is used: two 10-mm ports laterally and one 5-mm port in the midline. The lateral ports are placed approximately one-third of the way between the anterior superior iliac spine and the umbilicus, and the midline port is placed approximately 2–3 cm above the pubis, using the same precautions (transillumination and visual inspection for vessels) as for standard transperitoneal laparoscopic techniques (Figs 4.9 and 4.10). The midline trocar, followed by the right lower quadrant trocar are typically placed first to allow easy blunt dissection of the left side of the pelvis prior to placement of the left lower quadrant trocar. After the trocars are placed, the pressure should be decreased to 8–10 mmHg. Care is taken to assure that the lateral trocars are not placed through the peritoneum. Should the peritoneum be opened, it is very difficult to complete the procedure extraperitoneally. In this event, the trocars are placed intraperitoneally and a standard transperitoneal node dissection is performed.

The anatomical landmarks for the preperitoneal lymphadenectomy are identical to those of the standard open modified pelvic lymphadenectomy. The symphysis pubis and bladder can be identified in the midline and the pubic bone can be followed laterally on each side to identify the deep inguinal rings. The external iliac artery pulsations are also easily identifiable. The modified obturator pelvic lymph node dissection, normally performed at the time of radical retropubic prostatectomy, is used. This is a technique familiar to most urologic surgeons. The limits of the dissection are proximally the bifurcation of the iliac vessels, distally the circumflex iliac vein to include the lymph node of Cloquet, laterally the lateral border of the external iliac vein and posteromedially the obturator nerve.

The operating surgeon stands on the contralateral side to the dissection and the patient is placed in slight Trendelenburg and rotated towards the

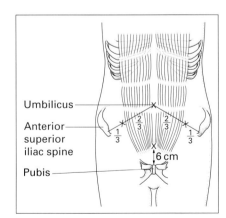

Fig. 4.9 Sites for trocars for the extraperitoneal lymphadenectomy are generally similar to the transperitoneal approach.

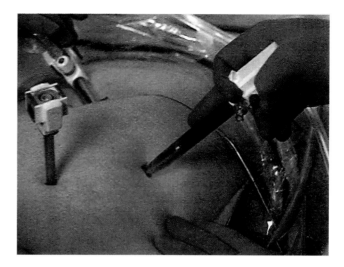

Fig. 4.10 Standard trocar placement techniques are used (inspection for vessels and transillumination).

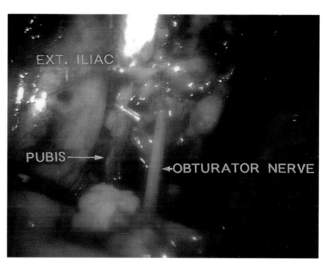

Fig. 4.11 An example of a completed left-sided dissection. It is identical to the final result of an open surgical approach.

surgeon. The procedure is begun by an incision in the fibroareolar tissue along the medial side of the external iliac artery. Blunt medial dissection identifies the external iliac vein and defines the lateral edge of the nodal package. The vas deferens is typically seen crossing obliquely and can be clipped and divided if needed. Dissection is performed along the external iliac vein, developing the lymph node package both proximally and distally. At the distal edge of the packet, careful dissection is carried out to identify any accessory obturator vessels, which are clip ligated.

The obturator nerve is identified at the posteromedial border of the dissection. The nodal package is dissected proximally as one piece off the obturator fossa and nerve. The exposure can be optimized by using a laparoscopic vein retractor on the external iliac vein. At the intersection of the obturator nerve and the iliac vein, blunt and sharp dissection are used to develop the proximal extent of the nodal package, with clips being used to seal the proximal lymphatics. Removal of the package is accomplished by the use of large grasping forceps through a 10/11-mm trocar sheath. The obturator fossa is irrigated and carefully inspected for haemostasis. The completed dissection is shown in Fig. 4.11. The identical procedure is repeated on the other side.

Before exiting the preperitoneal space, the pressure is lowered to 5–6 mmHg to ensure that no bleeding is being tamponaded by the higher pressure. At the end of the procedure, the trocar sheaths are removed and the fascial defects of the 10-mm ports are closed with 0 Vicryl or Dexon sutures. The gas is allowed to escape through the Hasson cannula, and the scrotum is manually decompressed if there is evidence of pneumoscrotum. The umbilical fascial defect is closed by tying the two pre-placed stay sutures, but the fascia must be carefully examined to confirm proper fascial closure. The wounds are irrigated with saline and the skin is approximated using a 4/0 undyed Vicryl or Dexon subcuticular running suture. The nasogastric tube is removed.

Results

We have recently reported on our initial experience of extraperitoneal pelvic lymphadenectomy using the trocar-mounted balloon device [19]. Extraperitoneal pelvic lymph node dissection with PDB was successfully accomplished in 12 of our initial 16 patients. The last eight consecutive procedures have been completed successfully. Three patients were converted to open pelvic lymph node dissection for intractable intra-operative hypercarbia, inadvertent entry into the peritoneal cavity and inadequate exposure of the external iliac vessels. One further patient was converted to the transperitoneal laparoscopic approach because of entry into the peritoneal cavity. Further analysis of patients who were converted to open surgery or a transperitoneal approach revealed that two had had prior hernia repair and one had a history of a ruptured appendix. The fourth patient, who experienced intra-operative hypercarbia, had a history of chronic obstructive pulmonary disease (COPD) and mild coronary artery disease. Based on our experience, we currently consider a history of prior hernia surgery, appendectomy or other groin or lower abdominal procedures to be a relative contraindication to the extraperitoneal laparoscopic approach.

For the successfully completed extraperitoneal approach the mean (with standard deviation) estimated blood loss was 65±15 ml, the mean operative time was 146±31 minutes and the mean node count 8±4. Post-operatively, patients were allowed to begin eating on the night of surgery and the Foley catheter was removed when the patient was alert and ambulating. All 12 patients who were successfully operated extraperitoneally were discharged within 24 hours, returned to full activity in a week and had no post-operative complications. In one patient a 3-cm asymptomatic lymphocoele was discovered on a repeat staging magnetic resonance imaging (MRI) following a course of neoadjuvant therapy.

Advantages and disadvantages

There are several theoretical and practical advantages of the extraperitoneal laparoscopic approach. The open (Hasson) technique is used routinely for the extraperitoneal approach, thus eliminating the complications related to the blind insertion of a Veress needle or initial trocar (such as perforation of a viscus, vascular injury or gas embolism). The reduced insufflation pressure is beneficial in reducing complications related to barotrauma and adverse cardiovascular effects. The chance of a serious electrocautery injury to a visceral organ is virtually eliminated. By avoiding the peritoneal cavity, the risk of visceral and vascular injury during surgical dissection may be reduced and the preperitoneal landmarks, such as Cooper's ligament and the iliac vessels, can be visualized directly. Intestinal retraction may be easier since the 'peritoneal envelope' surrounds the intestines and therefore individual bowel loops need not be retracted. The operating time may also be decreased and prolonged post-operative ileus might be less common due to less intestinal retraction and manipulation, and the fact that the colon does not need to be mobilized. In addition, this approach may reduce the potential risk of seeding of tumour cells or bacterial contamination of the peritoneal cavity, and fluid collections such as urinoma or haematoma may be more easily contained. Shoulder pain caused by intraperitoneal CO_2 should be eliminated, and there is also a suggestion that herniation through the trocar sites and post-operative bowel obstruction may be reduced, with less post-operative adhesions compared with the transperitoneal approach. Finally, the extraperitoneal approach to the node package is a very familiar technique to surgeons performing radical retropubic prostatectomy.

The extraperitoneal approach does have some limitations and disadvantages. Prior abdominal surgery may render this technique difficult or even impossible. In obese patients, excessive fat may obscure the extraperitoneal anatomy. Excessive fat is less of a problem when performing a transperitoneal node dissection. The working space is limited and smaller than the peritoneal cavity, which may make intracorporeal suturing, organ entrapment and removal more difficult and time-consuming. Since there is no cleaning surface such as intestine on which to clean the lens, the visibility may be affected and in this situation the self-cleaning Hydro-laparoscope (ACMI, Stamford, Connecticut, USA) may be more helpful. Inadvertent entry into the peritoneal cavity will obliterate the extraperitoneal space with insufflation, and the surgeon may need to convert to the standard transperitoneal approach or even to open surgery. Another disadvantage of this approach for pelvic lymphadenectomy is that it may render subsequent radical retropubic prostatectomy more difficult due to the development of extraperitoneal adhesions. One more disadvantage of this technique is balloon rupture, although the newer manufactured devices are more reliable and less prone to breakage. However, if a balloon does rupture careful inspection is needed to assure that no fragments are left behind.

Although it has been suggested that hypercarbia is less with the extraperitoneal approach, the literature is not clear on this point, and absorption of CO_2 may actually be greater in the extraperitoneal space than it was originally thought. Wolf and co-workers [20] recently reported greater absorption of CO_2 in retroperitoneal versus transperitoneal nephrectomy, as well as a greater incidence of pneumothorax and pneumomediastinum. No patient in their series, however, had any sequelae of hypercapnia, which was easily managed by aggressive ventilation. There have been reports of refractory hypercarbia with both intra- and extraperitoneal techniques, and the relative absorptive capacities of the peritoneum and extraperitoneal space may not be significantly different under the influence of CO_2 insufflation. The potential advantages of the extraperitoneal approach in this regard need to be more thoroughly investigated as more experience is gained with this technique.

McDougall and co-workers [21] have compared their initial 20 patients, who had undergone transperitoneal procedures, to six subsequent patients who underwent retroperitoneal laparoscopic nephrectomy. The transperitoneal group had a somewhat shorter operative time (5.8 hours vs. 6.7 hours), required more analgesics post-operatively (30mg morphine sulphate vs. 14mg), had a longer convalescence (12 days vs. 9 days) and suffered more complications (4 vs. 1) than the retroperitoneal group. However, total hospital stay was similar (4 days) in both groups. Based on this initial experience, the authors concluded that although the retroperitoneal approach may be technically more demanding, it results in fewer complications and less post-operative morbidity than the transperitoneal approach.

Gasless laparoscopy

Recently, the gasless extraperitoneal technique has been used to perform pelvic lymphadenectomy. Albert and Raboy [22] have utilized this technique successfully in 16 patients with prostate cancer, and we have used the technique in a number of extraperitoneal pelvic procedures [23]. The surgical technique is basically the same as described above for the EPLND, the only difference being that an external retraction system is employed rather than CO_2 insufflation. The Laparofan–Laparolift system (Origin Medsystems, Menlo Park, California, USA), a commercially available retraction system, is used to maintain the working space (Fig. 4.12). After performing the 'open laparoscopy' technique described above and developing the extraperitoneal space using balloon dissection, the Laparofan (a fanlike retractor) is inserted through a valveless trocar placed in the initial infraumbilical incision site, connected to the Laparolift (a motorized retraction system) and retracted to provide a working space (Fig. 4.13). The remainder of the procedure is performed as described above. This retraction system permits controlled abdominal wall retraction to produce an adequate laparoscopic working cavity. Proper positioning of the Laparolift at the beginning of the procedure is important to prevent its interference with movements and transfer of laparoscopic instruments. The telescope design of the arm and the rotational feature of the Laparofan permit vertical retraction with the blades pointing in any direction. The opened fan retractor elevates the abdominal wall in a planar direction, and the motorized electromechanical Laparolift arm has a self-regulator that can control the power of retraction to any predetermined level. A distinct advantage of this system is that a variable degree of abdominal lift can be tailored to the particular needs of the procedure and can be adjusted to the length requirements of standard surgical instruments, decreasing the costs of expensive laparoscopic instruments. In addition, this system can allow for digital palpation and tactile feedback via the trocar incision, and facilitates extracorporeal knot tying and suturing techniques because a pneumoperitoneum does not have to be maintained.

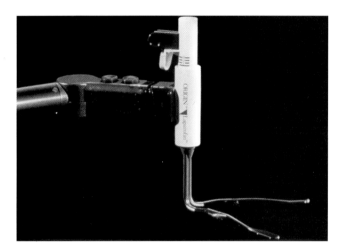

Fig. 4.12 The Laparolift system (Origin Medsystems, Inc., Menlo Park, California, USA) for gasless laparoscopy.

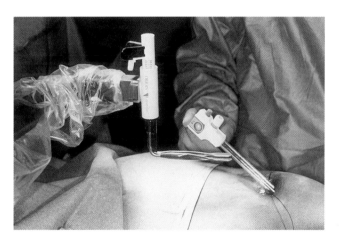

Fig. 4.13 The Laparolift ready to be positioned in the extraperitoneal space.

With the obvious advantages of avoiding complications related to CO_2 insufflation and the ability to use standard surgical instruments, the gasless technique offers potential advantages as an alternative laparoscopic technique. However, the gasless technique still has some technical drawbacks for pelvic urological procedures. Although it can provide adequate working space, the exposure can be limited, especially for the more proximal portions of the dissection since there is a tendency for the peritoneal envelope to rise up with each breath. Further refinements are underway of both the device and the procedure.

Conclusions

Many of the complications associated with the traditional transperitoneal laparoscopic approach can be avoided by controlled distension of the extraperitoneal space using the PDB.

The use of a motorized retraction system for the gasless technique has the advantages of avoiding the complications associated with CO_2 insufflation and allowing the use of standard surgical instruments. Further work is being done to improve the exposure during pelvic lymphadenectomy and at present the gasless approach should be regarded as investigational.

Extraperitoneal laparoscopy is an exciting modification to standard transperitoneal laparoscopy. Its versatility is limited only by the skill and imagination of the surgeon and it is likely that many more laparoscopic urological procedures will be performed through this approach in the future.

References

1 Winfield HN, Donovan JF, See WA *et al.* Urological laparoscopic surgery. *J Urol* 1991; 146: 941–948.
2 Abdel-Meguid TA, Gomella LG. Complications of laparoscopy: prevention and management (unpublished observations).
3 Freiha FS, Salzman J. Surgical staging of prostate cancer: transperitoneal versus extraperitoneal lymphadenectomy. *J Urol* 1977; 118: 616–617.
4 McCullough DL, McLaughlin AP, Gittes RF. Morbidity of pelvic lymphadenectomy and radical prostatectomy for prostate cancer. *J Urol* 1977; 117: 206–207.
5 Grossman IC, Carpinello V, Greenburg FH, Malloy TR, Wein AJ. Staging pelvic lymphadenectomy for carcinoma of the prostate. *J Urol* 1980; 124: 632–634.
6 Steiner MS, Marshall FF. Mini-Laparotomy staging pelvic lymphadenectomy (minilap). Alternative to standard and laparoscopic pelvic lymphadenectomy. *Urology* 1993; 41: 201–206.
7 Gomella LG, Albala DM. Laparoscopic urological surgery. *Br J Urol* 1994; 74: 267–273.
8 Gomella LG, Abdel-Meguid TA, Hirsch IH *et al.* Laparoscopic urologic surgery: continued improvement in outcome. *J Urol* 1995; 153: 358 [abstract].
9 Hald T, Rasmussen F. Extraperitoneal pelvioscopy: a new aid of staging of lower urinary tract tumors. A preliminary report. *J Urol* 1980; 124: 245–248.
10 Ferzli G, Trapasso J, Raboy A, Albert P. Extraperitoneal endoscopic pelvic lymph node dissection. *J Laparoendosc Surg* 1992; 2: 39–44.
11 Ferzli G, Raboy A, Kleinerman D, Albert P. Extraperitoneal endoscopic pelvic lymph node dissection vs. laparoscopic lymph node dissection in the staging of prostatic and bladder carcinoma. *J Laparoendosc Surg* 1992; 2: 219–222.
12 Ferzli G, Raboy A, Albert P. Extraperitoneal endoscopic pelvic lymph node dissection. *Surg Endosc* 1994; 8: 124–126.
13 Hasson HM. Open laparoscopy: a report of 150 cases. *J Reprod Med* 1974; 12: 234–238.

14 Goldstein DS, Winfield HN. Laparoscopic instrumentation. In: Gomella LG, Kosminski M, Winfield HN, eds. *Laparoscopic Urologic Surgery.* New York: Raven Press, 1994: 32–33.

15 Gaur DD. Laparoscopic operative retroperitoneoscopy: use of a new device. *J Urol* 1992; 48: 1137–1189.

16 Keizur JJ, Tashima M, Das S. Retroperitoneal laparoscopic renal biopsy. *Surg Laparosc Endosc* 1993; 3: 60.

17 Coptcoat MJ, Eden CG. Laparoscopic retroperitoneal surgery. In: Coptcoat MJ, Joyce AD, eds. *Laparoscopy in Urology.* Oxford: Blackwell Scientific Publications, 1994: 110–120.

18 Gerber GS, Rukstalis DB, Chodak GW. The role of laparoscopic lymphadenectomy in the staging and treatment of urological tumors. *Ann Med* 1993; 25: 127–129.

19 Gomella LG, Lotfi MA, Abdel-Meguid TA, Moreno JG, Hirsch IH. Extraperitoneal laparoscopic lymphadenectomy using a trocar mounted balloon device (unpublished observations).

20 Wolf JS, Monk TG, McDougall EM *et al.* The extraperitoneal approach and subcutaneous emphysema are associated with greater absorption of CO_2 during laparoscopic renal surgery. Presented at the 12th World Congress of Endourology and ESWL, St. Louis, 1994, abstract P5–145.

21 McDougall EM, Clayman RV, Fadden PT. Retroperitoneoscopy: the Washington University Medical School experience. *Urology* 1994; 43: 446–452.

22 Albert PS, Raboy A. Extraperitoneal endoscopic 'gas-less' pelvic lymph node dissection. *Current Surgical Techniques in Urology* 1994; 7: 5.

23 Hirsch IH, Moreno JG, Lotfi A, Gomella LG. Noninsufflative laparoscopic access. *J Endourol* 1995; 9: 483–486.

5 Colposuspension

R. J. S. HAWTHORN

The traditional abdominal approach to colposuspension in the management of genuine stress incontinence has used extraperitoneal dissection to reach and identify the bladder neck before suturing the vagina at the level of the bladder neck to the iliopectineal ligament. The classical Burch colposuspension is one of the procedures which produces the best long-term results [1]. The extraperitoneal laparoscopic approach described below closely mimics the traditional open operation.

Preparation and planning

Careful patient selection and counselling prior to the procedure includes confirming the diagnosis of genuine stress incontinence by urodynamic testing if the best results are to be obtained. The results of other pre-operative investigations should be available, such as electrocardiogram (ECG), chest X-ray and full blood count, if thought appropriate. The general contraindications to laparoscopic surgery should be considered before contemplating this approach.

Preparation for surgery commences in the clinic. The patient should be advised that if the procedure is completed laparoscopically then a short post-operative hospital stay of the order of 36–48 hours is likely. She should be encouraged to ensure that sufficient help at home is available for the initial post-operative period, enabling her to cope with day-to-day needs. She should also be made aware that a rapid recovery towards normal activities is expected and should be encouraged. There would seem to be little point in undertaking laparoscopic colposuspension for the patient who was not well motivated and keen to make the most of her rapid recovery. The patient should be advised that an indwelling suprapubic catheter will be *in situ* initially and there may be a possibility of early discharge from hospital with the catheter *in situ*. This requires a policy of catheter management to be agreed with those concerned, i.e. nursing and medical staff. Our policy will be discussed later.

The patient should be fasted from midnight on the evening before surgery if this is planned in the morning. Fasting from 6 a.m. may be acceptable for afternoon procedures.

It is essential that the operator is properly organized in terms of both time and equipment. The theatre list should be planned accordingly; a minimum of 2 hours should be allowed for the first attempted case. When laparoscopic suturing is planned it is highly desirable that the operator has practised the technique in the laboratory beforehand. He or she should have some idea of which needle holder is best suited for the task to be performed, which sutures are to be used and the type of knots to be tied.

Any equipment to aid vision and definition is most helpful when suturing and a 3-chip-type camera with a high-definition TV monitor are desirable. The progression of 3-D video technology may considerably improve this area but at present this technology is almost prohibitively expensive. Other than the equipment mentioned above, laparoscopic extraperitoneal colposuspension involves little else other than mounted gauze pledgets and laparoscopic scissors to cut sutures.

Anti-embolic stockings are routinely employed in our department, although prophylactic heparin is not usually given for laparoscopic procedures. The suprapubic hair should be shaved to allow the abdominal ports to be placed as low as possible.

Consent

Following admission the procedure should be explained to the patient, preferably by the operator. The operator should ideally present the results of his or her own experience. Consent should include permission to open the abdomen and complete the procedure should intra-operative problems be encountered.

Positioning and preparation of the patient in theatre

The patient's legs should ideally be placed in Lloyd-Davis stirrups with the hips only slightly flexed and a generous Trendelenburg tilt employed. The bladder should be emptied and a Foley catheter left *in situ* with the balloon distended with 10–20 ml of sterile water to allow easy identification of the bladder neck. The catheter should then be connected to a bag of saline from which 200 ml has been removed, and then left on continuous drainage. An ampoule of methylene blue should be added to the depleted bag of saline. At any time during the procedure the bag can be elevated to fill and define the bladder. This is particularly useful should a bladder perforation be suspected. A bimanual examination should be undertaken before surgery to confirm no gross pelvic abnormalities and reasonable vaginal mobility and capacity.

Distending the extraperitoneal space

The difficulty with the extraperitoneal approach to colposuspension is finding this space in a logical, consistent and safe manner. Various techniques are described to facilitate this, from balloon distension devices to optical trocars. Some even have balloons integrated into optical trocars. Open laparoscopy using a Hasson-type approach may also be used. In our experience the simplest and most direct method has proven to be the best.

The pubic symphysis should be palpated and a Veress needle inserted about one finger breadth above and angled towards the middle of the back of the symphysis pubis. The tactile sensation is similar to placing the Veress needle intraperitoneally and often a 'pop' is also heard as the needle passes through the rectus sheath and tendinous insertion of the rectus muscles. As there is no posterior rectus sheath at this level, the Veress needle is now in the cave of Retzius, which is a low-pressure space similar to the peritoneal cavity and distends easily. This insertion should be below the site of any previous surgery.

Carbon dioxide (CO_2) is insufflated at 1–2 l/min with a preset pressure of 12–15 mmHg. The Foley catheter should be draining freely into the bag of saline. Since the bladder is the only viscus likely to be perforated with this low insertion of the Veress needle this will be easily recognized if the bag of saline distends with gas.

Placement of the primary trocar

An intraumbilical incision is made in the usual fashion. The initial approach has been modified recently to use an optical trocar (Visiport, United States Surgical Corporation, Norwalk, Connecticut, USA; Fig. 5.1) instead of a reusable trocar to allow the operator some visual control over the placement of the primary trocar. The laparoscope is placed in the optical trocar and the near focus adjusted. The blunt trocar is then tunnelled subcutaneously above the rectus sheath from the umbilical insertion to half-way between the umbilicus and pubic symphysis in the midline. The trigger handle of the Visiport activates a small blade and with the trocar now directed almost vertically through the rectus sheath the fibrous tissue of the rectus sheath is cut in small portions by the blade of the Visiport. Continuous pressure has to be applied to the trocar and with repeated cuts the trocar advances through the sheath and muscle into the cave of Retzius. This process is easily followed as the sheath appears very white, with the muscle beneath looking red. As soon as the

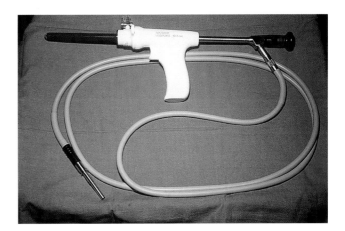

Fig. 5.1 The Visiport (United States Surgical Corporation, Norwalk, Connecticut, USA) with laparoscope inserted.

muscle has been traversed the trocar is in the cave of Retzius. The trocar and laparoscope are now removed leaving the 10-mm cannula *in situ*. The laparoscope is now reinserted. Most gynaecologists have found themselves in the cave of Retzius at some time inadvertently during routine laparoscopic surgery. The appearance of the 'spider's web' of filmy 'adhesions' is instantly recognizable to most.

Dissection in the cave of Retzius

The initial dissection is performed by the CO_2. The tip of the laparoscope can also be used to perform some dissection if it is advanced onto the symphysis pubis and gently moved from side to side. The laparoscope may be palpated through the abdominal wall to confirm its position on the symphysis pubis.

A 5-mm trocar can then be inserted in the midline, replacing the Veress needle. This marks the position of the midline and allows scissors or grasping forceps to be inserted and dissection of the loose tissue in the cave of Retzius to be completed before the two lateral trocars are inserted. The symphysis and both iliopectineal ligaments should be easily identified at this stage.

Placement of secondary trocars

The lateral cannulae are inserted 4–5 cm from the midline, one on each side at the same level or slightly more cephalad than the initial 5-mm port (Fig. 5.2). The dissection of the cave of Retzius should be sufficient to enable the site of entry of the lateral ports to be clearly seen. The ideal site may be estimated by attempting to place the lateral cannulae in the abdominal wall directly over the part of the iliopectineal ligament where the sutures are to be placed. Indenting the abdomen whilst observing the laparoscopic view from the cave of Retzius is very valuable.

The author prefers to use 10-mm cannulae laterally to allow easy passage of a gauze pledget mounted on grasping forceps (Fig. 5.3), which is used to complete the dissection and mobilize the bladder. If such a system is employed, it is essential that a suture be passed through the pledget and the end left long enough to emerge from the port, enabling easy retrieval of the pledget in the event that it becomes dislodged from the grasping forceps. Other operators may prefer to perform the dissection with scissors and in these circumstances 5-mm ports may suffice, particularly if disposable peanut-type pledgets are used.

The choice of metal or plastic cannulae is also important since metal cannulae with their sharp edges tend to abrade and cut through the sutures, often very easily. For this reason the author now prefers to use plastic cannulae through which to suture. The type produced by Dexide (Atlantic Medical, Glasgow, UK) have the added advantage that the splaying and locking mechanism retracts some tissue out of the way and ensures that only about 1 cm of the cannula actually projects into the cave of Retzius. Since the cannula is fixed to the abdominal wall it does not

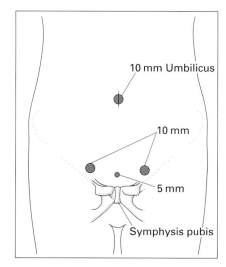

Fig. 5.2 Port sites and sizes.

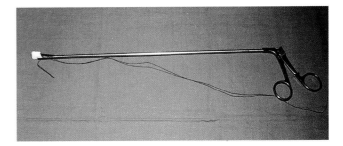

Fig. 5.3 A gauze pledget mounted in grasping forceps with a long suture secured to the pledget.

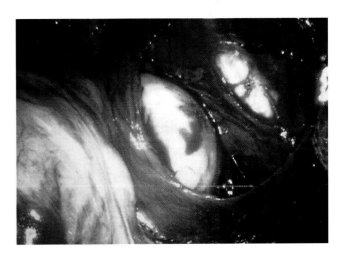

Fig. 5.4 The right iliopectineal ligament is displayed. The white fibres of the vagina are seen with the operator's finger elevating the vagina. The bladder lies on the left.

become dislodged during the procedure and can even be used to elevate the abdominal wall if necessary.

Mobilization of the bladder neck

Using the mounted pledget, the iliopectineal ligament on the first side to be sutured should be clearly displayed by removing any fatty or loose areolar tissue from the area of the iliopectineal ligament through which the sutures are to pass (Fig. 5.4). The fibres of the ligament should be identified before the bladder is mobilized, and with the magnification and clear vision possible using the laparoscopic approach any particular vascular areas are easily avoided. This should be performed on one side at a time as some slight bleeding may be encountered. Being right-handed, the author finds it easiest to display the right iliopectineal ligament first with the grasping forceps and gauze pledget passed through the ipsilateral port.

The bladder neck is then identified with the help of the Foley catheter balloon and the bladder mobilized medially from the vagina at this level using the pledget and a gentle pushing motion. This is most easily performed with the operator's own left index finger elevating the vagina from below whilst an assistant guides the laparoscopic procedure. Mobilization is complete once the white fibres of the vagina are visible, as in the open Burch procedure.

Suturing of the vagina to the iliopectineal ligament

With the vagina and iliopectineal ligament clearly visible, suturing is commenced. The nature of suture material, number of sutures to be used on each side, and type of needle and needle holder are determined by the individual preferences of the operator. 'J'-shaped needles tend to be difficult to manipulate laparoscopically. Curved needles of any size are easily passed through the 10-mm cannulae or by using the back-loading technique described by Reich and colleagues [2]. They are readily manipulated with a little experience but are easily bent, especially if the pubic bone is encountered. It is not difficult to imagine that the needle will break in some circumstances once attempts at straightening have been made. 'Fixed-position'-type needle holders allow easier manipulation and suturing with curved needles but have no flexibility if the needle requires fine repositioning (Fig. 5.5). It has been our practice to use non-absorbable sutures and to place two sutures on each side at open colposuspension. This practice, combined with the comments above and much

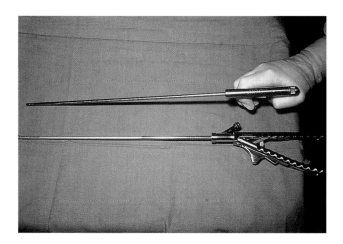

Fig. 5.5 Fixed-position needle holder is shown above with the more traditional type below.

experimentation, has led the author to use Ethibond on a straight needle (Ethicon EX 10G, Ethicon, Edinburgh, UK) and a simple traditional-type needle holder to place two sutures on each side.

The straight needle is grasped through the ipsilateral port. It is then dropped onto the bladder, grasped and orientated to about 90° to the needle holder before being passed through the vagina (Fig. 5.6). The needle is re-grasped at an angle of about 45° to the needle holder with the point directed towards the handle of the needle holder. The operator's finger in the vagina allows the needle manipulations to be made with some tactile sensation. The medial border of the iliopectineal ligament should be palpated with the needle holder to confirm that the suture is to be placed as high as possible. The needle holder is drawn upwards, thus driving the needle through the medial aspect of the iliopectineal ligament from below to above the ligament (Fig. 5.7). The suture is then withdrawn through the ipsilateral port and knotted extraperitoneally using a modified Roeder knot. This knot is then pushed down with the vagina

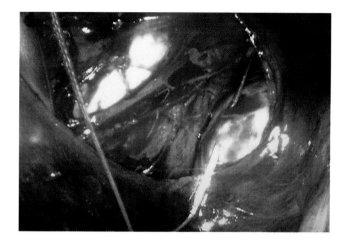

Fig. 5.6 Suturing technique. The suture is first passed through the vagina on the right.

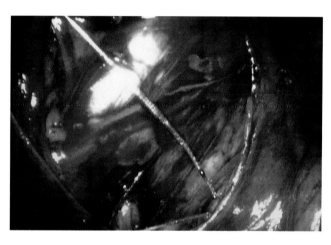

Fig. 5.7 Suturing technique. After being passed through the vagina the suture is then passed through the iliopectineal ligament.

elevated, now with the assistant's finger, to the iliopectineal ligament and the suture cut.

The suture described above has an integral knot pusher attached and this simplifies the procedure. However, half hitches may be tied and pushed down the cannula using a reusable instrument, such as the Clark–Reich knot pusher. Indeed, it is advisable to have this type of instrument available since occasionally the suture may break or the integral pusher not function effectively. Intracorporeal suturing is not performed since it is difficult to complete the knots securely.

A 'dog ear' of vagina is thus created (Fig. 5.8) and this makes placing the second suture very simple. The needle is passed through the desired part of the 'dog ear' and iliopectineal ligament (Fig. 5.9) before being tied and cut as described above (Fig. 5.10). The procedure is then repeated on the other side, commencing with exposure of the iliopectineal ligament. Each suture has to be placed, tied and cut individually, unlike the open procedure, as multiple threads are very confusing and get in the way of the laparoscopic instruments.

Other techniques avoiding laparoscopic suturing have been described. It is possible to staple mesh to the vagina and iliopectineal ligament to effect elevation. Other operators have placed the suture through the

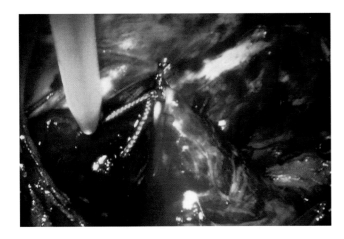

Fig. 5.8 Suturing technique. The knot is tied and pushed down with the integral knot pusher creating a 'dog ear'.

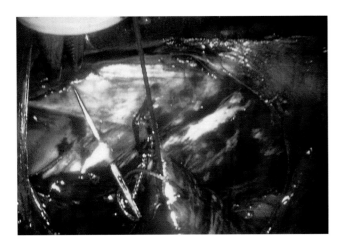

Fig. 5.9 Suturing technique. The second suture is passed through the 'dog ear' and through the iliopectineal ligament.

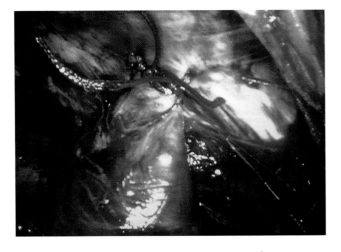

Fig. 5.10 Suturing technique. The suture is cut to complete the first side.

vagina and then secured the suture to the iliopectineal ligament using staples before the knot is tied [3]. Another recent development has been the introduction of a disposable suturing device (EndoStitch, United States Surgical Corporation, Norwalk, Connecticut, USA), which some operators may prefer at added expense.

Completing the procedure

Once all four sutures are in place the bladder is filled by elevating the bag containing methylene blue and its integrity checked. The 5-mm central cannula is removed and a suprapubic catheter inserted under direct vision through the skin incision and into the filled bladder. A suction drain can then be placed through one of the lateral cannulae if necessary.

The wound sites are then closed in two layers and the Foley catheter removed before the patient is returned to the recovery ward.

Post-operative care and catheter management

It is our usual practice to use a patient-controlled analgesia (PCA) system for pain relief. This was initially employed to enable an easy comparison of analgesic requirements between women having open and laparoscopic colposuspension.

Patients are encouraged to mobilize as early as possible and are commenced on 5 days of oral Co-amoxiclav as prophylaxis against urinary tract infection. Anti-embolic stockings are routinely employed in theatre and for the duration of the hospital stay.

The suprapubic catheter is left on free drainage until 10 p.m. on the day following surgery. It is then clamped and the residual volume checked the following morning. A further residual volume is checked at lunchtime on the second day and the catheter removed, and the patient discharged, if both measured volumes are less than 100 ml.

The women are aware, from pre-operative counselling, that if their bladder is not emptying satisfactorily they may be discharged with the suprapubic catheter *in situ*. In such cases the women are shown how to check their own residual volumes and are told to contact the ward when two consecutive measurements are satisfactory.

All patients are encouraged to contact the ward rather than their general practitioner should they experience any immediate post-operative problems following their discharge from hospital.

All women, where possible, are seen one week later at the clinic to check residual volume and voiding function.

Results, outcome and comments

Initial results indicate that with experience the operating time reduced towards a level comparable with open colposuspension. In our hands the time has been reduced from 150 minutes to under 30 minutes for the uncomplicated case. The median blood loss recovered in suction drains was 25 ml in 48 hours initially. The amount of intra-operative bleeding is significantly less than at open colposuspension. This is probably due to the tamponade effect of the pressure of CO_2 on the small vessels near the bladder neck. Since vision is considerably improved at laparoscopy less trauma and mobilization of the bladder is required, thus further reducing intra-operative bleeding (Table 5.1). Such is the dramatic reduction in intra-

Table 5.1 Extraperitoneal laparoscopic colposuspension.

Disadvantages
Operating time
Insufflating cave of Retzius
Laparoscopic suturing
Repair of bladder perforation
(Previous bladder neck surgery)

Advantages
Good visibility in cave of Retzius
Anatomy easily defined
Little bleeding
Reduced analgesia requirements
Reduced time to normal voiding
Reduced hospital stay
Rapid recovery to normal activities
Good short-term results

operative blood loss that diathermy and suction irrigation are virtually never required.

Even in the first 10 cases the suprapubic catheter was able to be removed at 48 hours in all but one patient, enabling early discharge. The median amount of PCA used in 48 hours was 21 ml, equivalent to 21 mg diamorphine. Three weeks was the average time to resumption of normal daily activities (Table 5.1). No urinary tract infections were recorded and no patient requested an emergency call from her general practitioner. Wound infections have not been recorded.

Short-term urodynamic follow-up using the subjective test of a visual analogue score and objective pad test confirms a very satisfactory outcome at 6 months. Maximum flow rates post-operatively are reduced and maximum voiding pressures increased, suggesting the obstructive element needed to achieve a good result is present following laparoscopic colposuspension (Table 5.2).

These encouraging initial results prompted a randomized trial to compare the described laparoscopic extraperitoneal technique with the open Burch colposuspension. Longer-term follow-up of over 70 patients has shown two patients in the laparoscopic group with subsequent detrusor instability, which compares favourably with those having the open Burch procedure. In total three cases have been converted to open procedures because of a trocar injury to the bladder early in the series and because of peritoneal entry at the start of one procedure, which made vision in the cave of Retzius very limited. The last case was converted to an open Burch colposuspension before any incisions had been made because of anaesthetic difficulties. Only one procedure has failed on longer-term follow-up of 6 months, with the others being cured or at least significantly improved.

Table 5.2 Outcome following laparoscopic colposuspension.

	Pre-operative	Post-operative
Visual analogue score (cm)	7.75 (2.5–10)	0.3 (0–7)
Standardized pad test (g)	16.1 (2–45)	0 (0–10)
Maximum flow rate (ml/s)	25.0 (14–43.2)	17.3 (6.9–21.9)

Results expressed as median with range.

Even in the initial series previous surgery, including hysterectomy, vaginal repair and caesarean section, were not considered to be contra-indications to undertaking laparoscopic colposuspension. A previous low transverse scar, particularly following hysterectomy, may make easy distension and recognition of the cave of Retzius difficult and occasionally the peritoneum may be entered. Should this occur, the procedure is likely to be prolonged as the peritoneum may balloon up and limit vision in the extraperitoneal space. However, with patience, it should be possible to complete the procedure. Marked obesity has not proven to be a significant problem when using the laparoscopic approach: our heaviest patient to date weighed in excess of 90 kg. Laparoscopic surgery has not been undertaken in women who have had any previous failed surgical attempts to treat their stress incontinence. The advantages and disadvantages of the technique are summarized in Table 5.1.

Additional minor intraperitoneal laparoscopic surgery is possible using the port placement described above if the cannulae are advanced through the peritoneum on completion of the colposuspension. Access is, however, compromised to some extent. If hysterectomy or other significant intraperitoneal laparoscopic surgery is planned then a transperitoneal approach for the colposuspension is best [3–5]. The secondary trocars are also introduced into the peritoneal cavity before the dissection proceeds over the dome of the bladder to enter the extraperitoneal space. The disadvantage of this approach is that it converts an otherwise extraperitoneal procedure into an intraperitoneal operation with additional risks to large vessels, especially the inferior epigastric vessels, and to the other intraperitoneal viscera. In the presence of known or suspected intraperitoneal adhesions, and particularly when there is a history of significant pelvic or abdominal surgery, the additional risks of entering the peritoneum are avoided with the extraperitoneal approach. Since the transperitoneal approach also involves abdominal dissection to gain access to the extraperitoneal space the operating time tends to be prolonged and the risk of bladder perforation is increased. Injury to the bladder at this part of the procedure is to the dome and although this is easily repaired laparoscopically if necessary, the repair is also time-consuming. An exclusively extraperitoneal procedure avoids the risk of bowel herniation and removes the need to close the port site fascia. Lastly, if laparoscopic surgery is to become acceptable as an alternative to conventional abdominal colposuspension, an attempt should be made to make the laparoscopic procedure as similar as possible to the original if results are to be compared and long-term follow-up with randomized trials conducted.

Long-term studies comparing open with laparoscopic colposuspension are needed to confirm the benefits of this approach to the management of genuine stress incontinence. Employing the objective tests of urodynamic measurement will allow a real comparison of operative results and it is our aim to follow our trial patients for at least 2 years.

References

1 Jarvis JJ. Surgery for genuine stress incontinence. *Br J Obstet Gynaecol* 1994; 101: 371–374.
2 Reich H, Clarke HC, Sekel L. A simple method for ligating in operative laparoscopy with straight and curved needles. *Obstet Gynecol* 1992; 79: 143–147.
3 Lyons TL. Minimally invasive retropubic colposuspension. *Gynaecol Endosc* 1995; 4: 189–194.
4 Vaincaillie TG, Schuessler W. Laparoscopic bladder neck suspension. *J Laparoendosc Surg* 1991; 1: 169–173.
5 Liu CY. Laparoscopic retropubic colposuspension. *J Am Assoc Gynecological Laparoscopists* 1993; 1: 31–35.

6

Inguinal herniorrhaphy

C. J. VAN STEENSEL & R. U. BOELHOUWER

Inguinal hernia repair is one of the most frequently performed operations in the Western world. It is interesting to note that from the time of Caspar Strohmeyer's monograph on inguinal hernia surgery in the 15th century there were no significant advances in hernia surgery until Bassini described his technique for repair in 1884 [1]. However, even this technique did not reduce the recurrence rate to a truly acceptable level; in as recent a period as 1977–89, the proportion of recurrent hernia repairs performed in The Netherlands in males >20 years old was 15–18%. Although this percentage is lower for females (8–10%), it is still arguably too high [2].

The first technique for endoscopic hernia repair, the 'plug and patch' repair published in 1990, was soon abandoned due to its high recurrence rate [3]. Although the prosthetic repair described by Stoppa [4] is associated with a lower recurrence rate, it failed to become popular because of the greater dissection necessary to perform it and its consequent higher morbidity. However, recent advances in technology have presented the opportunity of combining the low morbidity of minimal access surgery with the low recurrence rate of the Stoppa technique. This has led to a noticeable trend away from transabdominal techniques towards the more logical and easier to perform total extraperitoneal procedure (TEP).

Preparation and positioning of the patient

After induction of anaesthesia with muscle relaxation and endotracheal intubation, the patient is positioned supine on the operating table. A urinary catheter is unnecessary if the patient voids immediately before premedication. Prophylactic antibiotics are not routinely administered.

Unilateral hernia repair

Establishing an extraperitoneal workspace

A 1–1.5 cm transverse incision is made at the lower umbilical crease and the anterior rectus sheath exposed by blunt dissection. This is incised transversely over 1–1.5 cm from the linea alba towards the side of the hernia, allowing access to the plane between the rectus abdominis muscle and its posterior sheath, by separating the muscle fibres in the midline.

A transparent balloon trocar containing a 0° laparoscope is introduced into this plane (Fig. 6.1). The trocar is then advanced towards the symphysis pubis by gentle manipulation. At the level of the semicircular fold of Douglas, where the posterior rectus sheath terminates, it enters the preperitoneal space (Fig. 6.2). The correct position of the balloon is confirmed visually after inflating it with a small volume of air. Further insufflation of the balloon is then performed until the pubic bone is visualized or until insufflation produces no further dissection, which is a sign of impending balloon rupture (Fig. 6.3). The balloon trocar is replaced by a locking trocar to prevent gas leakage. The preperitoneal space is maintained with CO_2 insufflated to a maximum pressure of 15 mmHg. The umbilical port is used as the camera port (Fig. 6.4).

Placement of secondary ports

A second trocar is introduced under endoscopic vision in the midline halfway between the umbilicus and the symphysis pubis (Fig. 6.5). The peri-

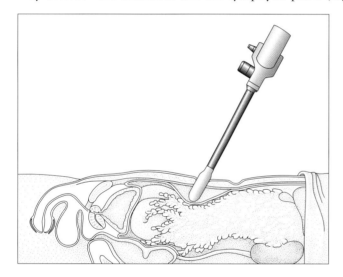

Fig. 6.1 The preperitoneal plane is entered through a sub-umbilical incision and a balloon trocar is introduced.

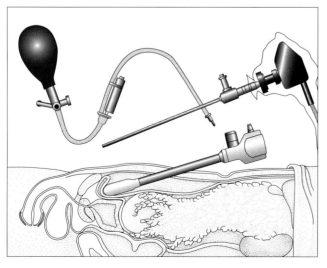

Fig. 6.2 The balloon trocar is advanced through the preperitoneal plane. The laparoscope has not yet been inserted.

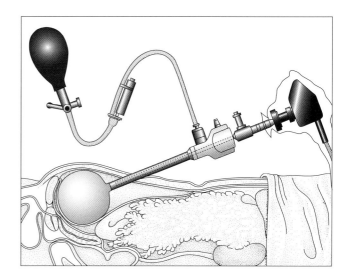

Fig. 6.3 The balloon, with the laparoscope inserted, is insufflated, allowing creation of a preperitoneal workspace under vision.

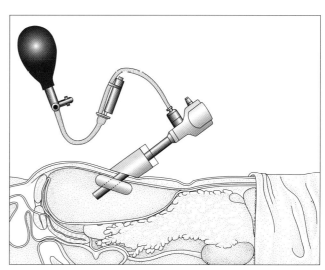

Fig. 6.4 A trocar preventing leakage of gas is inserted and the preperitoneal workspace is insufflated with CO_2 at a maximum pressure of 15mmHg.

toneum in the same lower abdominal quadrant as the hernia is swept off the tranversalis fascia by blunt dissection and a third trocar is inserted at the level of the umbilicus. At least one of the secondary ports must be 10mm in diameter to allow insertion of the mesh prosthesis.

Dissection of the hernia sac

The hernia is located by following the line of the inferior epigastric vessels. The contents of a direct hernia are easily reduced by traction on its contents, medial to the inferior epigastric vessels bordering Hesselbach's triangle. Reduction of an indirect hernia is more difficult as care must be taken to preserve the contents of the spermatic cord. The dissection of the sac of a large scrotal hernia may be particularly difficult. In this instance, transection of the hernial sac and closure of the peritoneal defect, leaving the sac *in situ*, may be the only option. After freeing the hernial sac from its adhesions to the abdominal wall and cord structures the deperitonealization continues until the extent of dissection extends horizontally from the symphysis pubis to the lateral trocar and caudally to intersect an imaginary line drawn from the lower edge of the superior pubic ramus to a point 5 cm below the lower edge of the internal inguinal ring (Figs 6.6 and 6.7).

The repair

The basis of this technique is the tension-free closure of the defect in the abdominal wall using a polypropylene mesh. The 15 × 10-cm mesh is tightly rolled and then inserted into the preperitoneal space through a 10-mm port (Fig. 6.8). The unrolled prosthesis is positioned so that it covers the femoral and inguinal hernial orifices, and extends from the midline to the lateral trocar, including the internal ring, Hesselbach's triangle and the superior pubic ramus (Fig. 6.9). Although staple fixation of the prosthesis has its proponents, the authors prefer to rely on intra-abdominal pressure alone to ensure that the mesh remains in place in most cases. If the mesh refuses to lie correctly, staples can be used but must not be placed along the lower rim of the mesh in the area between the vas and the testicular vessels because of the danger of injuring the external iliac artery. The other danger area, in which the lateral cutaneous nerve of the thigh is at risk from staple placement [5], lies lateral to the testicular vessels. At the end of the procedure, the preperitoneal space should be desufflated under vision to confirm correct placement of the mesh.

Post-operative care

Most young, fit patients can be discharged from hospital within the first 10 hours following herniorrhaphy. There is no restriction on the resumption of normal daily activities, including carrying weights.

Results

The performance of any hernia repair technique needs to be measured in terms of analgesic requirement, complications and long-term recurrence rate. As the TEP was developed in 1993, the results of only a small number of studies are currently available to assess this technique. Although there are several studies in progress comparing laparoscopic with open herniorrhaphy, most of these compare the results of trans-peritoneal laparoscopic hernia repair with its open counterpart. The only completed large study comparing the TEP with conventional repair is the COALA (Conventional Anterior Repair versus Laparascopic repair) study [6].

The operative technique used in the TEP is certainly more technically demanding than in transperitoneal laparoscopic repair, but the results of both are very dependent on operator experience. This is well illustrated by the fact that in a large series reported by experienced surgeons

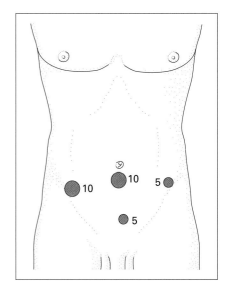

Fig. 6.5 Port sizes and sites.

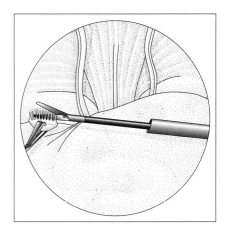

Fig. 6.6 Adhesions between the peritoneum and transversalis fascia are divided during deperitonealization of the left lower abdominal quadrant.

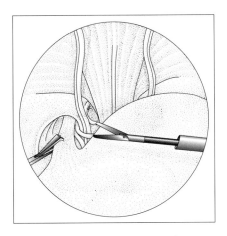

Fig. 6.7 The hernia sac of a left indirect inguinal hernia is reduced.

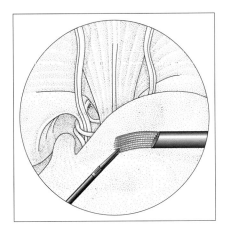

Fig. 6.8 The polypropylene mesh is introduced into the preperitoneal space through a 10-mm port.

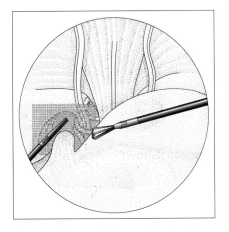

Fig. 6.9 The mesh is unrolled and positioned.

the operating times in the laparoscopic and open groups were not significantly different [6] and there appeared to be little learning-curve effect [6,7].

Analgesic requirement

At up to 6 weeks following surgery, post-operative discomfort as assessed by visual analogue scales and analgesic consumption was lower in patients undergoing the TEP compared with their open surgical counterparts [6]. These patients also resumed normal daily activities, including sport, sooner than those operated on by conventional means [6]. Physical performance tests in the early post-operative period, including straight-leg raising and sit-ups, yielded superior results in the laparoscopic group [8,9].

Complications

As in all methods of hernia repair, injury to the spermatic cord will occur in a small number of cases. Whilst venous bleeding is a commoner source of morbidity in open surgery, bleeding from epigastric or testicular arterial injury is commoner laparoscopically.

Endoscopically placed prosthetic mesh can become infected, but this is thankfully rare. One patient in our series developed such an infection which resulted in an abscess diagnosed by ultrasound (Fig. 6.10). This was successfully treated by ultrasound guided percutaneous drainage and antibiotic therapy. At 2 years' follow-up the patient still has no sign of recurrent infection or herniation.

Recurrence rate

There was no statistically significant difference in recurrence rate between the open and TEP groups, but there was a trend towards a lower rate in TEP-treated patients [5]. Within this group, most recurrences occurred in one centre, re-inforcing the influence of the learning-curve effect and individual surgeons' skills on results. Improved familiarity with the procedure, in conjunction with the fact that most recurrences in the TEP group occurred within the first year (compared with the continued recurrence rate in the conventional group), may translate into a significant difference in favour of the TEP in coming years.

Although the operating theatre costs associated with TEP are greater than those for open repair, these are usually offset by the lower post-operative analgesic requirement and the earlier return to work in these patients.

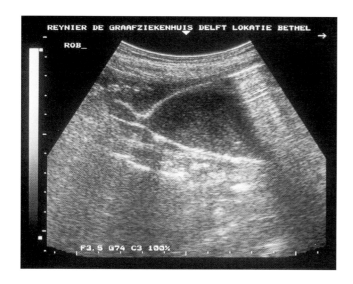

Fig. 6.10 Ultrasound scan of a polypropylene mesh prosthesis within an abscess cavity.

Bilateral hernia repair

Surgical approach

The approach for bilateral herniorrhaphy is merely an extension of that used for unilateral hernia repair. After the repair on the first side has been completed, deperitonealization on the side of the other hernia allows insertion of a fourth port, which is placed opposite the third (Fig. 6.5).

The repair

Bilateral inguinal hernia repair can be accomplished by using a second 15 × 10 cm polypropylene mesh, placed as in a unilateral repair, which overlaps the first. An alternative method, which resembles that used in the Stoppa technique, is to use a larger tailored prosthesis (Fig. 6.11) placed so that the smaller rectangle lies in the cave of Retzius, the rest of the mesh easily covering both inguinofemoral areas.

Results

Currently there are few data available on the results of bilateral TEP. In a recent series of 35 patients treated with a single large mesh with short-term follow-up there was a single hernia recurrence [10]. Although there have been no prospective randomized studies comparing laparoscopic and open bilateral inguinal hernia repair, logic suggests that as conventional bilateral repair is associated with a greater morbidity than unilateral repair, the benefits of performing bilateral herniorrhaphy laparoscopically should be even greater.

The future

A definite answer to the question 'what is the best technique for inguinal

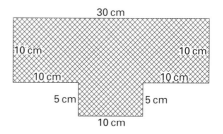

Fig. 6.11 Large mesh prosthesis for bilateral hernia repair.

hernia repair?' can clearly only come from a large prospective randomized trial. International co-operation would considerably ease this task and one such initiative is already underway in the form of ISLIR (International Study group in Laparoscopic Inguinal Hernia Repair), the results of which are awaited with interest.

Acknowledgements

We are grateful to AJM Karthaus for Figures 6.1–6.9.

References

1 Bassini E. Über die Behandlung des Leistenbruches. *Arch Klin Chir* 1890; 40: 429–476.

2 Dutch Centre for Health Care Information. *SIG Zorginformatie* 1994; Utrecht, The Netherlands.

3 Gerritsen A, van der Hoop G. *Laparoscopic Hernia Repair* 1994; thesis, University of Utrecht, The Netherlands.

4 Stoppa R, Moungar F, Henry X. Reparation des hernies de l'aine par grande prosthese de tulle de Dacron et voie d'abord pre-peritoneale. *Ann Ital Chir* 1993; 64: 169–175.

5 van Mameren H, Go PMNYH. Safe areas for mesh stapling in laparoscopic hernia repair. In Arregui ME, Nagan RF, eds. *Inguinal hernias, facts or controversies?* Oxford: Radcliffe Medical Press 1994, 483–487.

6 Liem MSL, van der Graaf Y, van Steensel CJ *et al*. A randomised comparison of conventional anterior and laparoscopic inguinal hernia repair. *N Engl J Med* (in press).

7 Liem MSL, van Steensel CJ, Boelhouwer RU *et al*. The learning curve for totally extraperitoneal laparoscopic inguinal hernia repair. *Am J Surg* 1996; 171: 281–285.

8 Liem MSL, van der Graaf Y, Zwart RC *et al*. A randomized comparison of physical performance following laparoscopic and open inguinal hernia repair. *Br J Surg* (in press).

9 Payne JH Jr, Grininger LM, Izawa MT *et al*. Laparoscopic or open inguinal herniorrhaphy? A randomized prospective trial. *Arch Surg* 1994; 129: 973–979.

10 Knook MTT, Weidema WF, de Graaf PW, van Steensel CJ. Endoscopic procedure for the Stoppa bilateral inguinal hernia repair. *Surg Endoscop* 1996; 10: 575.

7 Para-aortic lymph node sampling

J. J. G. BANNENBERG & D. W. MEIJER

The status of the para-aortic lymph nodes in patients with genitourinary malignancy has a significant impact on patient survival [1–3]. Lymph node status is also a key determinant in planning the extent of surgery or the field of radiotherapy. When the staging of these cancers is performed clinically, the outcome of these investigations is often inaccurate. In the case of carcinoma of the cervix, for example, there is a 30–40% discrepancy between clinical and surgical stage [2]. Sensitivity of lymphangiography is less than 30% [4]. Computed tomographic (CT) scanning and magnetic resonance imaging (MRI) are not sensitive enough if the nodes are not enlarged [4] and lymphoscintigraphy is too unreliable for routine use [5]. Fine-needle aspiration has a diagnostic accuracy of 74% [6]. When subclinical pelvic and/or para-aortic lymph nodes are not detected, the treatment field may be too small, resulting in reduced survival.

Although surgical staging allows for therapy to be tailored on a more scientific basis, resulting in an increased cure rate [1,2], the complications associated with para-aortic lymph node sampling using the traditional transperitoneal or extraperitoneal approaches are considerable. In the open surgical technique the extraperitoneal approach is preferred. Comparing both approaches, Berman found that the transperitoneal approach was associated with a 30% complication rate, following radiotherapy in the form of small-bowel damage. The extraperitoneal approach carried a 2.5% morbidity, due to small-bowel complications [7]. In many instances the small-bowel damage was segmental, and was found to have occurred in the areas where loops of small bowel were fixed to the posterior peritoneum by adhesions which followed a transperitoneal approach.

Endoscopic surgery has become, since the introduction of laparoscopic cholecystectomy, a popular alternative to the traditional approach in a variety of diseases. New developments in endoscopic technology and instrumentation allow access to the para-aortic lymph nodes that may decrease the morbidity of this surgical staging procedure.

In 1973 Wittmoser mentioned the possibility of para-aortic lymph node sampling as an indication for retroperitoneal endoscopy while performing a unilateral lumbar sympathectomy [8]. However, in 1991 Querleu stated that 'it is at this time impossible to explore the para-aortic nodes by laparoscopy' [9]. Shortly afterwards he and two other groups reported their first attempts at unilateral sampling of lymph nodes on the aorta, above the bifurcation and beneath the inferior mesenteric artery [10–12]. In 1993, Childers reported four cases of unilateral (two right- and two left-sided) high para-aortic lymph node sampling using a transperitoneal approach. In 1995 Coptcoat reported one case of removal through a total retroperitoneal approach of a single 3-cm residual mass beneath the left renal vein after chemotherapy for testicular cancer [13].

Para-aortic lymph node sampling

It is possible to use several different techniques for harvesting the retroperitoneally located para-aortic lymph nodes. As often seen with the development of procedures in laparoscopic surgery, a gradual learning curve can be observed in the attempts of the pioneers in this field. The most obvious route for the para-aortic lymph nodes in gynaecological and urological laparoscopy is the transperitoneal route, since most of the initial attempts to harvest these nodes were made in combination with other intra-abdominal procedures. This is also one of the limitations of the more direct extraperitoneal route to para-aortic lymph nodes.

Most standard techniques for low para-aortic lymph node dissection require, on the right side, dissection of lymphatic tissue over the vena cava from the level of the inferior mesenteric artery to the mid-common iliac artery. On the left side, this involves clearance of lymphatic tissue between the aorta and ureter from the level of the origin of the inferior mesenteric artery to the left mid-common iliac artery. Para-aortic node sampling in the staging of high para-aortic lymph nodes, as in ovarian carcinoma, must be extended to the level of the renal vein.

Technique of transperitoneal low para-aortic lymph node sampling

This technique has been described by various groups using a similar technique for the staging of endometrial [10] and cervical carcinomas [11]. Only the position of the ports is slightly different. The technique used allows access to the para-aortic lymph nodes below the level of the inferior mesenteric artery, as well as unilateral access to the common iliac nodes. A limiting factor is the inability to perform this procedure on patients weighing over 90 kg because of inadequate exposure of the para-aortic area [14].

The patient is put in a supine position with a 30–40° Trendelenburg tilt. Depending on the side of interest, the patient is also tilted to the left or right. A four-port technique is used: a 12-mm port at the umbilicus; two 5-mm ports midway between the umbilicus and the anterior superior iliac spines; and one 11-mm port in the midline a few centimetres above the pubic symphysis (Fig. 7.1).

The Trendelenburg position allows the intestines to be swept away from the operating field. An incision in the peritoneum overlying the right common iliac artery is made with scissors and extended superiorly. The

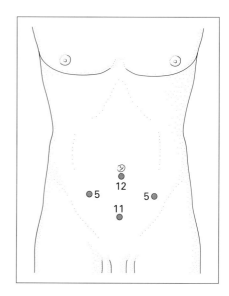

Fig. 7.1 Port position for transperitoneal low para-aortic lymph node sampling.

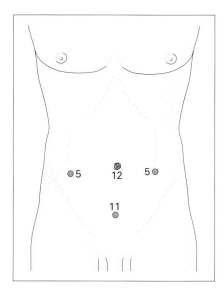

Fig. 7.2 Port position for transperitoneal high para-aortic lymph node sampling.

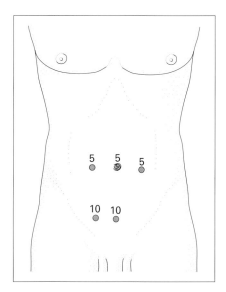

Fig. 7.3 Port position for transperitoneal high para-aortic lymph node sampling, as developed in a porcine model by Herd and co-workers.

peritoneum is retracted laterally to allow good visualization of the operating field.

Technique of transperitoneal high para-aortic lymph node sampling

The method published by Querleu [12] is a four-port technique in which the surgeon stands on the right and the assistant on the left of the patient. The patient lays in a supine, 15° Trendelenburg position, tilted slightly to the left. The first port in the umbilicus is for the laparoscope, operated by the assistant. Two 5-mm ports are positioned 10cm lateral to the umbilicus. The right one is manipulated by the surgeon's left hand, leaving the left one for retraction by the assistant. A fourth 10-mm port half-way between the pubis and umbilicus is used by the surgeon's right hand (Fig. 7.2).

Approaching from the right, the retroperitoneum is opened to expose the right common iliac artery and the lower aorta over 5cm, from its bifurcation to the origin of the inferior mesenteric artery. This approach allows lymph node sampling half-way down the common iliac arteries on both sides, both sides of the lower aorta up to the level of the origin of the inferior mesenteric artery, and along the right side of the vena cava up to the level of the right renal vein.

Querleu reported two cases of high para-aortic lymph node sampling using this technique for early ovarian carcinoma. Four patients were reported by Childers [15] with high unilateral para-aortic lymph node dissection for surgical staging of ovarian or fallopian unilateral carcinomas. For the two left-sided cases it was necessary to transect the left ovarian artery. One complication was reported: a hole in the vena cava which could not be controlled by pressure or clips and required laparotomy. It was not clear whether this was a patient in whom high or low para-aortic lymph nodes were sampled.

Herd and colleagues [16] described their laparoscopic transperitoneal approach in a porcine model for bilateral para-aortic lymph node sampling, using the peritoneum as a retracting sling with a five-port trocar technique (Fig. 7.3). Their dissection extended from the bifurcation of the right common iliac vessels to the renal veins. An incision in the peritoneum was made lateral to the right common iliac vessels and extended to the bifurcation of the aorta. The three 5-mm ports are used to retract the peritoneum via sutures that are attached to the dissected peritoneum. This does not prevent the use of other instruments through these ports at the same time. A grasper inserted through the middle 5-mm port is used for retraction. Depending on the position of the operator, the 10-mm ports are used for the laparoscope and scissors or clipping instruments. The operator handles the grasper through the middle 5-mm port and the instruments through the 10-mm suprapubic port. With this approach they succeeded in harvesting 88% of all para-aortic lymph nodes.

Technique of retroperitoneal high para-aortic lymph node sampling

A total retroperitoneal technique, as in open surgery, seems to be the most logical and direct approach to the para-aortic nodes. The technique used by Coptcoat [13] to remove a 3-cm chemotherapy-resistant nodal mass, consisted of a modified extraperitoneal laparoscopic nephrectomy approach. As a consequence, this technique is only suitable for unilateral sampling. The patient was positioned in the lateral position with the table fully broken. The port position is depicted in Fig. 7.4. Access to the retroperitoneum began with a 2-cm incision about 4 cm superior to the anterior superior iliac spine. Blunt finger dissection was used to create a space, following which retroperitoneal dissection was achieved using a Helmstein balloon. A 3-cm nodal mass on the left side was removed. Although the procedure was a success, 'it was clear that adequate visualization required medial displacement of surrounding structures and that any attempt to remove all post-chemotherapy lymphatic tissue would be

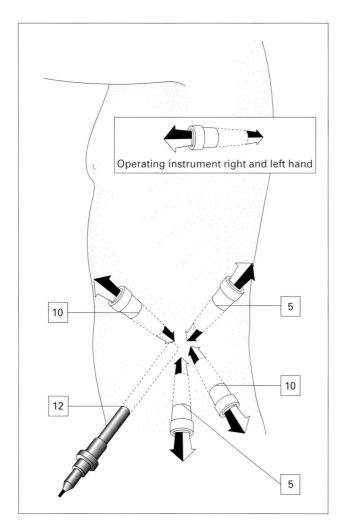

Fig. 7.4 Port position and sizes (in mm) for extraperitoneal laparoscopic para-aortic lymph node dissection. (From [13].)

very difficult given the instrumentation available and restricted angles of access.' [13].

The author's experimental prone technique of bilateral retroperitoneal para-aortic lymph node sampling

The author has described an experimental technique to sample lymph nodes on both sides of the aorta, using a porcine model to evaluate a retroperitoneal flank approach [17,18]. Animal position and port placement are demonstrated in Fig. 7.5. A subcutaneous patent blue 2% injection of 1–2ml is given between the toes in both legs to colour the lymph nodes.

Operative details

The surgeon sits on the left side of the animal, with the assistant on the surgeon's left to operate the camera. The creation of the preperitoneal space is done through a modified Hasson technique. Using the laparoscope as a blunt dissector, the preperitoneal space is further developed. Carbon dioxide (CO_2) pressure is maintained at 12mmHg. Once an adequate space has been created, a second 10-mm trocar is inserted 5cm to the right, dorsal to the first trocar. A third 10-mm trocar is placed 5cm to the left and dorsal to the initial trocar (Fig.7.5). These entry ports can help with the further dissection of the peritoneum towards the level of the aorta and the vena cava (Fig.7.6).

The aorta, the vena cava and their lymph nodes are identified, facilitated by the colouring of the lymph nodes with the patent blue. Dissection of the nodes lying between and on both sides of the large vessels begins at

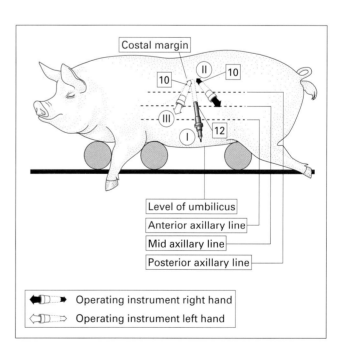

Fig. 7.5 Port position for para-aortic lymph node sampling in the prone position. (From [21].)

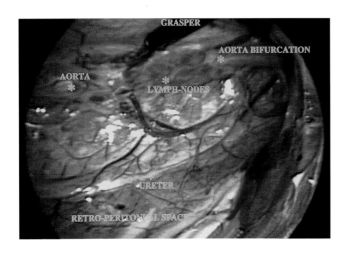

Fig. 7.6 Overview of the left retroperitoneal space: (clockwise from top) mid-para-aortic lymph nodes, aortic bifurcation, ureter and aorta.

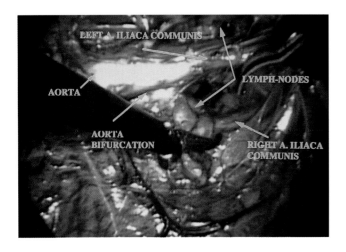

Fig. 7.7 Dissection of para-aortic lymph nodes from the left and right common iliac arteries and aortic bifurcation.

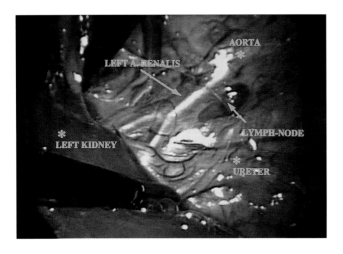

Fig. 7.8 View of the left retroperitoneal space with a lymph node on the left renal artery.

the aorta bifurcation, using this as a landmark, and extends to the level of the left renal artery (Figs 7.7 and 7.8). Dissection is continued using blunt grasping forceps and scissors connected to electrocautery.

After the laparoscopic procedure was concluded in the author's study a laparotomy was performed to identify any remaining para-aortic lymph nodes missed during the laparoscopic procedure.

Results

During the procedures performed there was no sign of injury to the peritoneum, the urinary tract, or the vascular structures in any of the pigs. In one pig, six para-aortic lymph nodes were removed laparoscopically. Subsequent laparotomy revealed an additional node. In the second and third pigs, seven and eight para-aortic lymph nodes, respectively, were removed endoscopically. Laparotomy failed to demonstrate any residual high common or pre-caval lymph nodes. Operation times for the laparoscopic procedures were 60, 50 and 45 minutes, respectively. Histological examination of the tissue proved that the specimens were indeed lymphatic tissue, as had been confirmed by the colouring of the tissue by patent blue.

Through a total retroperitoneal flank approach a good overview of both left and right high para-aortic lymph nodes was obtained. The lymph nodes were readily exposed once the preperitoneal pneumoperitoneum was achieved, thus minimizing the need for extensive dissection. Colouring the lymphatic tract contributed significantly to the identification of the lymph nodes. This specific technique also seems applicable to clinical cases [19]. Naturally, the situation in the porcine model is different from that in a human. The peritoneum is very thin and the area is relatively fat-free allowing for easy identification of the structures. Nevertheless, the prone position makes optimal use of the natural retraction of the intra-abdominal organs on the posterior peritoneum, providing an excellent view of the structures and eliminating the need for retraction. Viewing the abdominal anatomy in an upside-down position compared with normal surgery requires some adjustment but, as with any procedure, it becomes familiar after a few cases.

Following a transperitoneal approach the peritoneum is usually not closed or is only partly closed to allow drainage of lymph fluid. Although retroperitoneal drains were not placed in our reported cases, the use of a low-pressure vacuum drainage system is probably indicated [20], although the frequency of lymphocoele when using a totally retroperitoneal approach is unknown.

The disadvantage of retroperitoneal access is that it is technically more demanding in its creation than its transperitoneal counterpart, and that the created retroperitoneal working space is usually smaller. It is expected that in humans orientation will be more difficult because of the absence of familiar landmarks. Contraindications for transperitoneal endoscopic surgery, such as obesity, inadequate bowel preparation and intraperitoneal adhesions, are factors which might make the retroperitoneal approach more attractive.

The contribution that laparoscopic transperitoneal and retroperitoneal para-aortic lymph node sampling can make to the surgical staging of genitourological cancers needs to be determined by a wider experience with this technique in a prospective clinical study.

References

 1 Jones W. Surgical approaches for advanced or recurrent cancer of the cervix. *Cancer* 1987; 60: 2094–2130.
 2 Averette HE, Donato DM, Lovecchino JL, Seven B. Surgical staging of gynaecologic malignancies. *Cancer* 1987; 60: 2010–2020.
 3 Podczaski ES, Palombo C, Manetta A, *et al.* Assessment of pretreatment laparotomy in patients with cervical carcinoma prior to radiotherapy. *Gynecol Oncol* 1989; 33: 71–75.
 4 Vercamer R, Janssens J, Usewils R. Computed tomography and lymphangiography in the presurgical staging of early carcinoma of the uterine cervix. *Cancer* 1987; 60: 1745–1750.
 5 Feigen M, Crocker EF, Read J, Crandon AJ. The value of lymphoscintigraphy, lymphangiography and computer tomography scanning in the preoperative assessment of lymph nodes involved by pelvic malignant conditions. *Surg Gynecol Obstet* 1987; 165: 107–110.
 6 McDonald TW, Morley GW, Choo YC, Shields JJ, Cordoba RB, Naylor B. Fine needle aspiration of para-aortic and pelvic lymph nodes showing lymphangiographic abnormalities. *Obstet Gynecol* 1983; 33: 71–75.
 7 Berman ML, Lagasse LD, Watring WG, *et al.* The operative evaluation of patients with cervical carcinoma by an extraperitoneal approach. *Obstet Gynecol* 1977; 50: 658–664.
 8 Wittmoser R. Die Retroperitoneoskopie als neue Methode der lumbalen Sympathikotomie. *Fortschritte der Endoskopie* 1973; 4: 219–223.
 9 Querleu D, Leblanc E, Castelain B. Laparoscopic pelvic lymphadenectomy in the staging of early carcinoma of the cervix. *Am J Obstet Gynecol* 1991; 164: 579–581.
10 Childers JM, Surwit EA. Combined laparoscopic and vaginal surgery for the management of two cases of stage I endometrial cancer. *Gynecol Oncol* 1992; 45: 46–51.
11 Nezhat CR, Burrell MO, Nezhat FR, Benigno BB, Welander CE. Laparoscopic radical hysterectomy with paraaortic and pelvic node dissection. *Am J Obstet Gynecol* 1993; 166: 864–865.
12 Querleu D. Laparoscopic para-aortic node sampling in gynecologic oncology: a preliminary experience. *Gynecol Oncol* 1993; 49: 24–29.
13 Coptcoat MJ. Extraperitoneal pelvic and para-aortic lymphadenectomy. *Endosc Surg Allied Technol* 1995; 3: 9–15.
14 Childers J, Hatch K, Surwit E. The role of laparoscopic lymphadenectomy in the management of cervical carcinoma. *Gynecol Oncol* 1992; 47: 38–43.
15 Childers J, Hatch K, Tran A-N, Surwit E. Laparoscopic para-aortic lymphadenectomy in gynecologic malignancies. *Obstet Gynecol* 1993; 82: 741–747.
16 Herd J, Fowler JM, Shenson D, Lacy S, Montz FJ. Laparoscopic para-aortic lymph node sampling: development of a technique. *Gynecol Oncol* 1992; 44:271–276.
17 Bannenberg JJG, Meijer DW, Klopper PJ. The prone position; using gravity for a clear vision. *Surg Endosc* 1994; 8: 1115–1116.
18 Bannenberg JJG, Meijer DW, Klopper PJ. Extraperitoneal laparoscopic para-

aortic lymph node sampling in the prone position: development of a technique. *J Laparoendosc Surg* 1995; 5: 41–46.

19 Harzmann R, Hirnle P, Geppert M. Retroperitoneal lymph nodal visualization using 30% Guajazulen blue (chromolymphography). *Lymphology* 1989; 22: 147–149.

20 Heurn LWE, van Brink PRG. Prospective randomized trial of high versus low vacuum drainage after axillary lymphadenectomy. *Br J Surg* 1995; 82: 931–932.

21 Bannenberg JJG, Hodde KC, Hourlay P, Meijer DW. Experimental retroperitoneal endoscopic surgery. *Endosc Surg Allied Technol* 1995; 3: 21–26.

8 Lumbar sympathectomy

P. HOURLAY

Until recently, lumbar sympathectomy was reserved for the treatment of end-stage peripheral vascular disease with cutaneous ischaemia [1,2]. However, the adoption of a minimally invasive technique to perform the same operation offers the chance to broaden the indications to include the treatment of hyperhidrosis and the chronic lower limb pain of Sudeck's atrophy. Knowledge of the pathophysiology of these conditions and the increasing clinical experience in surgical endoscopy are the basis of this evolution.

First performed by Royle in 1923 for unilateral spastic paralysis of the leg [2,3], lumbar sympathectomy was also noted to produce capillary vasodilatation and local warmth. These phenomena form the rationale for the use of lumbar sympathectomy for the treatment of lower limb vascular insufficiency. However, sympathectomy not only causes relaxation of arteriovenous anastomoses, explaining the vasodilatation of the skin, but also causes an interruption of afferent pain pathways, making it a logical treatment option for Sudeck's atrophy.

Operative technique

The procedure is performed under general anaesthesia, using carbon dioxide (CO_2) to maintain the working space. Alternatively, the use of low-pressure CO_2 insufflation and an endoscopic mechanical retractor allows the procedure to be done under regional or local anaesthesia, but this is technically more demanding.

Patient position

The positioning of the patient on the operating table is identical to the position used for exposure of the kidney: the lumbotomy position with 45° lateral tilt. The table is broken at the level of the third lumbar vertebra (L3) (Fig. 8.1). This position provides the surgeon with a good endoscopic exposure, as well as allowing rapid open access to the peritoneal cavity and abdominal vessels if needed.

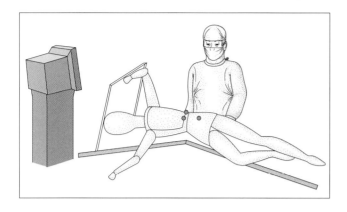

Fig. 8.1 Patient position.

Access

Digital dissection of the layer between the peritoneum and overlying muscle is performed through a 12-mm McBurney-type incision. This blunt dissection is developed laterally and posteriorly, along the psoas muscle. Use of the Visiport device (United States Surgical Corporation, Norwalk, Connecticut, USA), which incorporates a transparent cutting trocar, provides a very elegant alternative technique for entering the extraperitoneal space. Although created for accessing the peritoneal cavity under endoscopic control following CO_2 insufflation in patients with suspected intraperitoneal adhesions, this device may be used to create an extraperitoneal working space. After the Visiport has been introduced through an 11-mm surgical incision, the anterior fascia is cut and the muscle layer is split by pushing on the instrument. Insufflation of CO_2 through the trocar of this device then transforms the virtual space between muscle and peritoneal membrane into an actual working space. Care must be taken not to perforate the posterior fascia or the peritoneum. This manoeuvre, carefully done under endoscopic control, allows the rapid and safe creation of an extraperitoneal cavity through a limited skin incision. A purse-string suture should be placed through the skin and subcutaneous tissue to avoid CO_2 leakage around the cannula during insufflation.

Once the first port (either a blunt port or Visiport cannula) is in place (Fig. 8.2), CO_2 is insufflated at a rate of 2–10l/min with an upper pressure limit of 10–14mmHg.

Details of lumbar sympathectomy

Extraperitoneal blunt dissection is commenced using the laparoscope as a blunt dissector. This 'scope dissection' is performed parallel to the vertebral column on the medial aspect of psoas, at the sites of its insertion, and along its long axis (Fig. 8.3). In this way, the extraperitoneal cavity is progressively created. This gradual creation of the extraperitoneal space makes the procedure feasible even in patients who have undergone previous extraperitoneal surgery. Tilting the operating table to the opposite side is helpful. Dissecting along the long axis of psoas is an

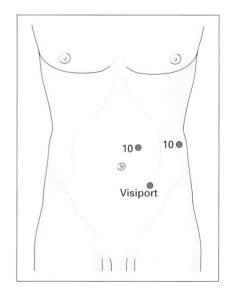

Fig. 8.2 Port placement.

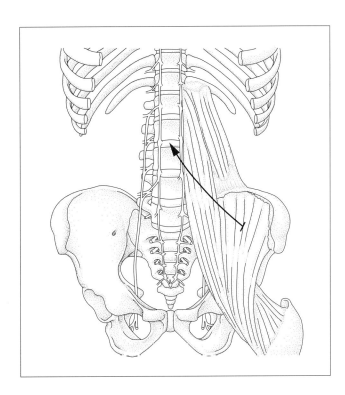

Fig. 8.3 Access to the left lumbar sympathetic chain.

important principle of this operation and enhances its reproducibility. It is also a useful method of locating and dissecting the major abdominal vessels, the ureter and the kidney.

A second 11-mm port is inserted under endoscopic control at the junction of the lumbar region and the flank, at the level of the umbilicus. The laparoscope is then transferred into this trocar.

A specially designed 10-mm dissector (Fig. 8.4) is introduced through the first port. In conjunction with the atraumatic retractor (Fig. 8.5), also designed by the author, this allows progress of the dissection along the abdominal aorta or vena cava and vertebrae. Under endoscopic control, a 5-mm port is placed at level L2–L3 in the umbilical region, at the medial

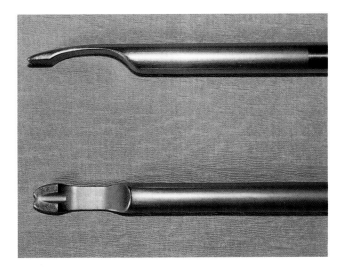

Fig. 8.4 Specially designed 10-mm blunt dissector.

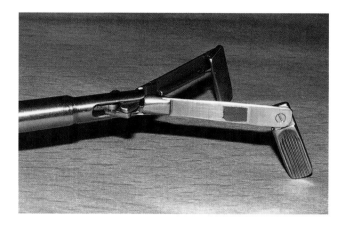

Fig. 8.5 Specially designed atraumatic retractor.

limit of the extraperitoneal dissection. Although other authors have advocated alternative port positions and commence their dissection more proximally, the positions used by the author result in better separation of the laparoscopic instrumentation.

An atraumatic grasper and shears with monopolar coagulation are introduced through the first and third ports. The sympathetic chain lies inside the insertions of the psoas muscle on the lumbar vertebral bodies. A gauze swab held by grasping forceps is used to visualize clearly the sympathetic chain (Fig. 8.6). The magnification of the laparoscope allows the surgeon to identify very accurately the anatomical structures. A segment of nerve fibres, including the L2–L3 ganglions, is excised (Figs 8.7(a)–(c)). A drain can be placed in the extraperitoneal cavity. In general this catheter is removed 24 hours post-operatively.

Results

Fourteen patients have undergone laparoscopic extraperitoneal lumbar sympathectomy, 12 for Sudeck's atrophy and two for end-stage peripheral vascular disease with cutaneous ischaemia. Eleven left-sided

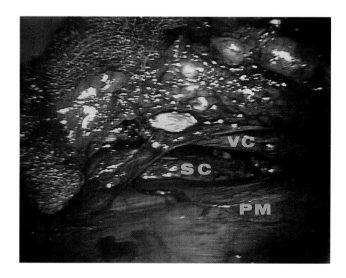

Fig. 8.6 Dissected right lumbar sympathetic chain (PM, psoas muscle; SC, sympathetic chain; VC, vena cava).

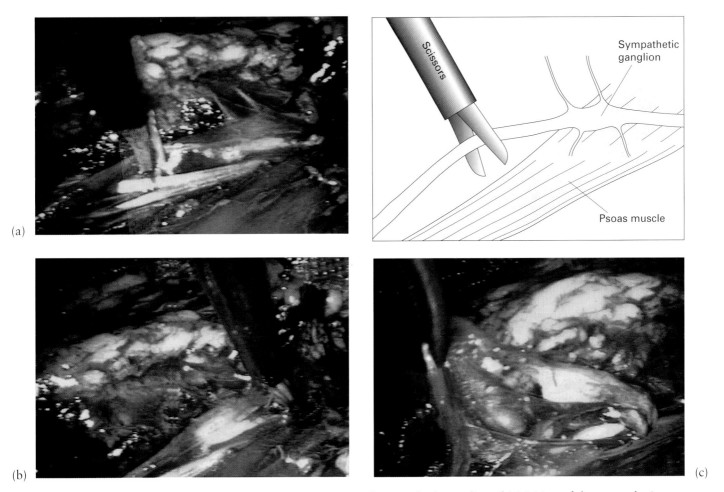

(a)

(b)

(c)

Fig. 8.7 (a) Dissected sympathetic ganglion. (b) Division of the sympathetic chain proximally. (c) The sympathetic chain is grasped and pulled caudally before excision.

and three right-sided sympathectomies were performed. One patient had previously undergone nephrectomy and an unsuccessful previous open sympathectomy on the same side.

The mean operating time was 38 minutes and the post-operative hospital stay was 2 days. In all cases, the clinical result was identical with the result of an open sympathectomy. No per- or post-operative complications were noted.

Potential complications

Perforation of the peritoneum reduces the extraperitoneal working space. It is possible to avoid this complication by using specially designed blunt dissectors developed to create the extraperitoneal cavity, decreasing the risks of peritoneal perforation. If a perforation in the peritoneum does occur, a Veress needle should be inserted into the peritoneal cavity to evacuate the intraperitoneal CO_2. The tension-free peritoneal membrane can then be closed using a clip.

During this dissection, great care must be taken not to traumatize the iliac vessels, ureter or gonadal vessels. Bleeding from lumbar vessels should be controlled by compression and/or clip placement.

The extraperitoneal endoscopic approach for lumbar sympathectomy appears to be as safe and as efficient as the open procedure but offers the advantages of minimally invasive surgery. The totally extraperitoneal approach avoids the need for intraperitoneal dissection, and the possibility of post-operative adhesions and shoulder pain.

References

1 Persson AV. Selection of patients for lumbar sympathectomy. *Surg Clin North Am* 1985; 65: 393–403.

2 Kissling R, Sager M. Morbus Sudeck—Erscheinungsbild und Therapie. *Unfallchirurgie* 1990; 16: 88–94.

3 Janoff KA, Phinney ES, Porter JM. Lumbar sympathectomy for lower extremity vasospasm. *Am J Surg* 1985; 150: 146–152.

9

Vascular applications, except sympathectomy

S. M. ANDREWS

Despite significant advances in endovascular therapies during the past decade, laparoscopy has had little impact on vascular surgical practice due to the perceived problem of achieving endoscopic surgical access and the potential for catastrophic bleeding. The difficulty of obtaining satisfactory access can be largely overcome by adopting the recently developed technique of balloon dissection [1], which can be adapted to create an extraperitoneal workspace in any part of the abdomen or pelvis. The problem of bleeding, which is inherent in any vascular procedure, is predictably more difficult to overcome. However, the magnification afforded by videoendoscopy has the potential to increase the accuracy of suture placement and thereby minimize anastomotic bleeding and promote long-term anastomotic patency.

Endoscopic approaches

Minimal access surgery to the abdominal aorta can be performed using either a transperitoneal or retroperitoneal approach.

Transperitoneal approach

Although most open intraperitoneal surgical procedures have been mimicked by laparoscopic surgeons, the dissection of retroperitoneal structures remains an enigma. This is especially so when the patient is in the supine position, due to the difficulty of retracting loops of intestine and to the fixity of their mesenteric attachment to the posterior body wall. An advantage of this approach is that access to the iliac vessels is very straightforward. Indeed, successful transperitoneal laparoscopic synthetic graft replacement of the iliac artery has been reported in a pig model [2].

Extraperitoneal approach

Balloon dissection of the retroperitoneum may be used to create an extraperitoneal workspace for minimal access vascular procedures, including dissection of the aorta. The technique of extraperitoneal laparoscopic aortic dissection has been developed in a porcine model by the author, but it remains an experimental technique at the time of writing. Although the procedure is relatively simple to perform in a porcine model, the initial learning curve is steep. The use of this laparoscopic approach avoids the difficulties of retraction of small-bowel loops, and post-operative adhesions between small-bowel loops and other structures, encountered in the traditional transperitoneal approach. Its chief disadvantage is that synchronous exposure of the iliac vessels is difficult and access to intraperitoneal viscera impossible.

Operative technique

Access is achieved using a standard open access balloon dissecting technique, as described in Chapter 2. A 10-mm laparoscopic port is inserted into the retroperitoneal space via the access wound and the wound edges sutured around it to prevent leakage of gas. Further ports are introduced into the space under direct vision, as required. For extraperitoneal laparoscopic aortic dissection two 10-mm and two 5-mm ports are recommended (Fig. 9.1).

The left kidney is identified, dissected and retracted medially, exposing the left renal artery and the aorta (Fig. 9.2), which are easily identified by

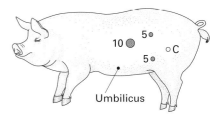

Fig. 9.1 Port placement for experimental extraperitoneal laparoscopic aortic dissection. Port sizes in mm. C, camera port (10 mm).

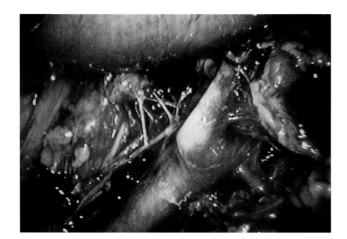

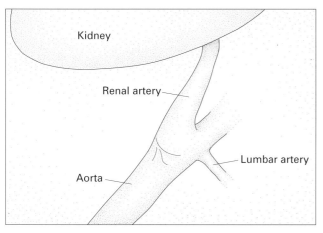

Fig. 9.2 Completed experimental extraperitoneal laparoscopic upper aortic dissection.

their pulsation. The aorta is then dissected superiorly and inferiorly as far down as the trifurcation by blunt and sharp dissection.

Care is needed to prevent tearing of the peritoneum during access, as the pneumoperitoneum leads to collapse of the retroperitoneal workspace. During dissection of the posterior aspect of the aorta the lumbar arteries should be carefully identified as avulsion may lead to haemorrhage and loss of view. Using this technique, an excellent view of the abdominal aorta, from above the renal arteries to the aortic trifurcation, can be obtained.

Experimental applications of extraperitoneal laparoscopic aortic dissection

Creation of an abdominal aortic aneurysm model

Current animal models of abdominal aortic aneurysm involve open exposure of the abdominal aorta and stripping of the media, insertion of a Dacron fusiform aneurysm or patch, or application of pharmacological agents to the aorta. However, open aortic dissection is traumatic and may induce physiological or pathological changes which could interfere with subsequent studies. Similarly, experimental aneurysms created by transluminal intimal application of agents such as elastase, require perfemoral access and may interfere with experiments requiring a subsequent perfemoral approach to the aorta, such as endoluminal stenting. Extraperitoneal laparoscopic exposure of the aorta overcomes some of these problems, providing a reproducible method of access to the adventitial surface of the aorta with the minimum of trauma.

Extraperitoneal laparoscopic aortic cross-clamping

Aortic occlusion is a necessary prerequisite to retroperitoneoscopic aortic procedures requiring aortotomy, such as prosthetic graft insertion, endarterectomy or patching, and angioscopy. Various minimal access manoeuvres are capable of achieving this, but the simplest involves inflation of a balloon within the aortic lumen. When performed via a femoral arteriotomy it has the disadvantage of precluding aortic stenting below the balloon, since the placement of the stent would entrap the balloon catheter. An alternative method involves aortic occlusion by an extraperitoneal laparoscopically placed sling or laparoscopic vascular clamp. Successful clamping is confirmed by the cessation of pulsation distal to the clamp. Aortotomy is performed following placement of proximal and distal aortic cross-clamps and placement of clips on the lumbar arteries, to prevent back-bleeding.

Aortic angioscopy

At present, aortic angioscopy is rarely practised due to the difficulty in gaining sufficient proximal vascular control to allow an adequate view.

However, following extraperitoneal laparoscopic aortic dissection and cross-clamping as described above, perfemoral angioscopy can be performed with a fine catheter inserted alongside the angioscope to flush blood from the aorta. This can be used to confirm the position and patency of previously placed stents and grafts.

Clinical applications

The clinical application of these techniques for the treatment of patients requiring surgical treatment of aneurysms is likely to be rather more difficult than its experimental counterpart, due partly to the presence of a greater amount of retroperitoneal fat in humans, but mainly to the significant difficulty inherent in dissecting an atherosclerotic, calcified and perhaps inflamed aorta.

The precise clinical utility of extraperitoneal laparoscopic aortic dissection is yet to be defined. Possible future roles include: (i) a prelude to abdominal aortic aneurysm sutured repair; and (ii) an adjunct to the endovascular treatment of aneurysms, allowing percutaneous aortic cross-clamping prior to endovascular exclusion of the sac, or by facilitating a combined angioscopic and retroperitoneoscopic sutured graft repair of abdominal aortic aneurysm.

References

1 Gaur DD. Laparoscopic operative retroperitoneoscopy: use of a new device. *J Urol* 1992; 148: 1137–1139.
2 Bessler M, Trokel M, Morales A, Treat MR, Nowygrod R. Laparoscopic vascular interposition graft. *Min Invas Ther* 1993; 2 (Suppl. 1): 89.

10 Ureterolithotomy

D. D. GAUR

Retroperitoneal laparoscopic ureterolithotomy was first performed in 1979 by Wickham [1] but did not assume popularity as the results of retroperitoneoscopy were uniformly poor. It was for the same reason that Clayman and co-workers performed an endoscopic ureterolithotomy by dilating a percutaneously established track under fluoroscopic control, and Meretyk and colleagues used a similar technique to remove a foreign body lodged near the ureter [2,3]. Attention was once again drawn towards the retroperitoneal laparoscopic approach to the ureter by Gaur in 1992 [4], who described a balloon technique for retroperitoneoscopy.

Indications

Retroperitoneal laparoscopic ureterolithotomy is indicated in a patient with a calculus anywhere in the ureter (except its intramural part) under the following circumstances: (i) when the calculus is large, hard or impacted; (ii) when extracorporeal shock-wave lithotripsy (ESWL) or endourological procedures have failed to retrieve the calculus; and (iii) when these minimally invasive facilities are either not available or not suitable for the patient.

Although a large, hard or impacted ureteral calculus could theoretically be treated by ESWL or endourological means, in practice this often entails multiple treatment sessions, requiring a prolonged hospital stay or repeat visits for retreatment. In addition to the possibility of increased morbidity as a result of the need for retreatment, there would be a greater chance of residual stone fragments at completion. Therefore, if the calculus is chronically impacted, larger than 15mm or larger than 10mm and hard, the author feels that it should be treated retroperitoneoscopically, as the whole calculus can be removed in a single sitting by this alternative minimally invasive technique. When deciding on the preferred mode of treatment for a patient with a ureteral calculus, one should bear in mind the fact that the more difficult a stone is to treat by ESWL or endourology, the easier it is to remove by retroperitoneoscopy [5].

Retroperitoneal laparoscopic ureterolithotomy can also be performed as a salvage procedure in patients where ESWL and endourological procedures have failed to render the patient stone-free. In developing countries, ESWL and endourological procedures are usually not available in government hospitals and the cost of treatment in private hospitals is prohibitively expensive for the average patient. Retroperitoneal laparoscopic ureterolithotomy is an economically viable procedure for these patients, as the laparoscopic equipment is usually freely available in most government hospitals as a result of family planning programmes.

Contraindications

Local inflammatory disease, a bleeding disorder or obesity are relative contraindications for retroperitoneoscopy. Severe cardiopulmonary disease, an aortic or an ipsilateral iliac artery aneurysm and dense retroperitoneal adhesions following inflammatory disease or previous surgery should be considered absolute contraindications for retroperitoneal laparoscopy, due to the high operative and balloon expansion risks in these patients. A thin patient with a large calculus impacted in the upper or mid-ureter is an ideal patient for the novice.

Pre-operative preparation

Informed consent

Informed consent must be obtained from all patients after explaining to them the risks, complications and the possibility of failure associated with any laparoscopic procedure.

Investigations

All patients should undergo routine investigations to assess fitness for anaesthesia and surgery. A urinary tract infection should be ruled out by urinary culture and an appropriate antibiotic given if required. Intravenous urography is mandatory in all patients and an ultrasound examination should also be carried out if any other retroperitoneal pathology is suspected. An immediate pre-operative plain X-ray of the abdomen should be carried out in all patients and, during the early part of the learning curve, this should be done with a coin strapped to the umbilicus to provide a landmark for the calculous bulge [6].

Medications

All medications affecting blood coagulation are stopped about a week earlier in consultation with the prescribing physician, but other medications are continued during the peri-operative period. Broad-spectrum antibiotics are given parenterally with the anaesthetic premedication. No bowel preparation apart from a simple enema is required.

Pre-operative procedures

A percutaneous nephrostomy drain should be established to prevent renal damage if hydronephrosis is associated with acute infection not responding to antibiotics. The infection should be allowed to subside before performing a retroperitoneoscopic ureterolithotomy to avoid the risk of post-operative septicaemic shock. Pre-operative insertion of an exdwelling ureteral catheter or guide wire helps in ureteral identification, but this may not be possible in all patients due to stone size and/or impaction. However, an open-ended ureteral catheter with a guide wire or a double J stent assembly advanced up to an impacted upper ureteral calculus helps not only in its identification, but also in post-operative placement of the stent. We do not use this technique routinely as it requires an extra procedure, is not cost-effective in our setting and identification of the ureter is not a major problem in our hands. Placement of a ureteral stent is reserved for patients in whom such a problem is anticipated due to obesity or inflammatory adhesions. A nasogastric tube is not required and an indwelling urethral catheter is inserted only for procedures on the lower ureter.

Anaesthesia

Cuffed endotracheal general anaesthesia is preferable to regional anaesthesia as it provides controlled muscle relaxation, which is crucial for a satisfactory pneumoretroperitoneum.

The operative procedure

The whole of the ureter can be exposed retroperitoneoscopically by using either a lumbar or iliac approach. The lumbar approach provides a good exposure of the upper and mid-ureter, while the iliac approach is equally good for the mid- and lower ureter. We have mostly used the lumbar approach in the past for both the upper and the mid-ureter, as it provides a better working space for endoscopic manipulation [7,8]. However, we now prefer the extended iliac approach (see Chapter 2) for the mid-ureter, as it provides a better exposure with a reasonably good working space.

The lumbar approach

The anaesthetized patient is placed in a lateral position and retroperitoneoscopy is performed, as described in Chapter 2.

ESTABLISHMENT OF ACCESSORY PORTS

Two accessory posterior ports are usually sufficient for retroperitoneoscopic ureterolithotomy, but a third anterior one may be required for retraction of the peritoneum and fat in some cases. The procedure can also be performed with a single secondary port in a select group of patients. The first port (10 mm) is placed posteriorly above the iliac crest, the second (5 mm) in the subcostal region at the posterior end of the marked kidney incision line, and the third (5 mm) anteriorly at the other end of the line (Fig. 10.1). For a calculus in the pelvic ureter, the size of the first and the second accessory ports should be reversed to allow use of a 10-mm endoknife, as described later in this chapter.

ALLOCATION OF PORTS

The first assistant manipulates the primary port instrument in the mid-axillary subcostal region, while the surgeon uses the posterior and the iliac ports for endoscopic dissection. The second assistant retracts through the anterior port if required. This port allocation allows the surgeon to sit comfortably throughout the procedure.

IDENTIFICATION OF THE URETER

If the balloon was placed deep to the fascia transversalis, the ureter can usually be identified over the reflected parietal peritoneum as soon as the laparoscope is inserted (Fig. 10.2). Even when the balloon has not been placed in the proper plane, it is not very difficult to locate a dilated ureter during endoscopic exploration. However, one should be wary of assuming that any tubular structure in that area is the ureter, as it is possible to mistake the gonadal vessels, inferior mesenteric vessels and even the inferior vena cava for the ureter. The upper ureter can also be identified by a stone bulge, if it is fairly large. If the ureter cannot be visualized

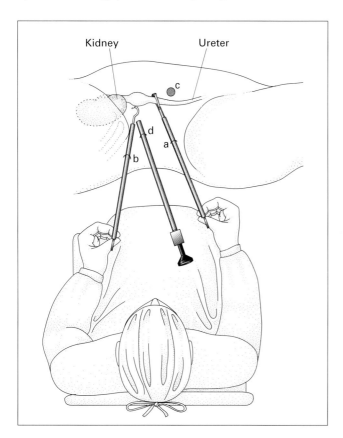

Fig. 10.1 The position and the orientation of the three commonly used ports for a right upper ureterolithotomy are shown. The surgeon can sit down comfortably and operate through the iliac (**a**) and the renal angle (**b**) ports, while the assistant standing to his right controls the primary port (**d**). The anterior port (**c**) is only rarely required.

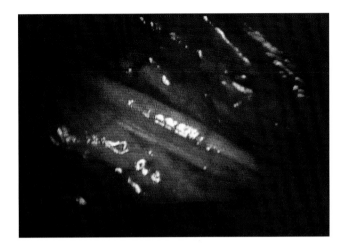

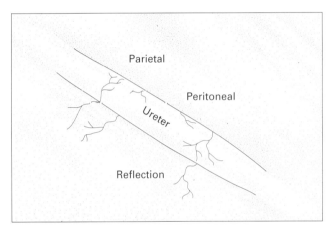

Fig. 10.2 The abdominal ureter, dissected by the balloon, is seen as soon as the laparoscope is inserted.

during preliminary retroperitoneoscopy it must be located by dissection, which can sometimes be time-consuming.

If the parietal peritoneum has already been adequately dissected, the ureter should be searched for posterior to the gonadal vein and anterior to either the aorta or inferior vena cava, depending on the side of the stone. Otherwise, it should be located by retracting the psoas and lifting up the parietal peritoneum with the convex surface of a 10-mm blunt spatula dissector. If this fails to locate the ureter, it should be searched for by palpating it with a 5-mm spatula dissector by repeatedly stroking it over the reflected peritoneum and the psoas from above downwards, right up to the iliac bifurcation [9]. When searching for the ureter near the lower pole of the kidney, it helps to make the ureter taut by lifting up the kidney. The use of a ureteral stent or illuminator [10] may be of great help in these patients.

DISSECTION OF THE URETER

No further dissection of the ureter is required if the stone-bearing part has been neatly dissected by the balloon. Otherwise, endoscopic dissection of the ureter must be performed until the stone bulge is clearly visible. Endoscopic dissection of the ureter can be performed with a single accessory port if the calculus is at L4 level and there is good dissection of the retroperitoneal space (Fig. 10.3). The second accessory port is only required for suturing the ureter in these patients. If the pneumoretro-peritoneum is not very satisfactory and the peritoneum and retroperitoneal fat keep falling down over the ureter, the third accessory port is established to allow the use of a retractor.

If the calculus is above the level of L4, the ureter is grasped with an endoBabcock forceps through the iliac port and is dissected proximally with the 5-mm spatula dissector through the other posterior port until the stone bulge is just visible. This is done by engaging the peri-ureteral fibroareolar tissue at the tip of the dissector and gently stripping it off the ureter (Fig. 10.3). Sharp dissection with endoshears is only required if there are dense peri-ureteral adhesions. As soon as the stone bulge is seen retrograde dissection of the ureter should be stopped to prevent the calculus from being dislodged. The ureter is grasped below the calculus with Babcock forceps to gently pull it down and the stone bulge dissected with a hook dissector in an antegrade direction (Fig. 10.4). The ureter is grasped just above the stone bulge with another Babcock after the stone-bearing ureter has been dissected. The first Babcock is then removed.

If the calculus is below L4 level, the dilated ureter is grasped with a

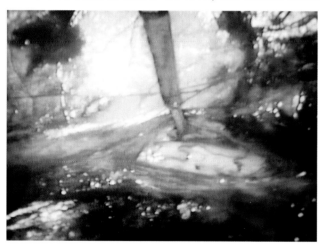

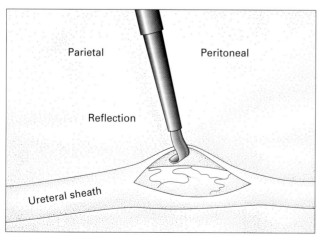

Fig. 10.3 The abdominal ureter is dissected from its sheath with a 5-mm spatula dissector through the iliac port.

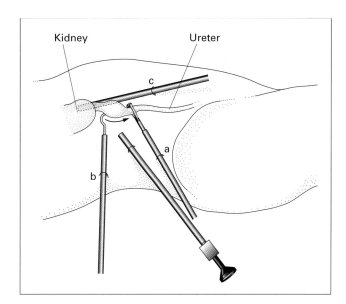

Fig. 10.4 The right upper ureter is grasped with Babcock forceps through the iliac port (**a**) just distal to the calculus. The stone-bearing ureter is dissected with a hook through the renal angle port (**b**) in an antegrade direction. The second assistant may be required to lift the lower pole of the kidney with a blunt 10-mm dissector through the anterior port (**c**).

Babcock through the posterior subcostal port and is similarly dissected down to the calculus. A calculus up to S2 level can be dissected using this approach by pushing the pelvic peritoneum medially using the Babcock which is holding the ureter. If the pneumoretroperitoneum is not satisfactory, the pelvic peritoneum should be retracted by the second assistant using a suitable retractor. The use of a 30° laparoscope might help during this dissection. Care must be taken when pulling the ureter off the pelvic wall to prevent an avulsion injury. When dissecting the upper right ureter and the lower left ureter the surgeon might have to cross hands, if he wants to avoid dissecting the ureter left-handed. Usually there is not much bleeding during the dissection of the ureter and electrocoagulation is rarely required. Localization of the calculus is usually easy but may occasionally be difficult if the stone bulge is inconspicuous. The calculus may even be seen through a dilated ureter if the latter is not inflamed. However, the position of the calculus in the ureter should always be confirmed by palpating it with fallopian tube-holding forceps. An ultrasound probe can help in a doubtful case, especially if the calculus has migrated unexpectedly.

INCISING THE URETER WHEN THE CALCULUS IS LOCATED IN THE UPPER URETER

The ureter is grasped proximal to the calculus with Babcock forceps through the posterior subcostal (renal angle) port and is gently pressed against the psoas to steady it for the incision through the iliac port (Fig. 10.5(i)). In a situation where the ports have to be crossed to allow use of the 10-mm endoknife, the Babcock is passed through the 5-mm iliac port, pressed against the psoas and rotated in such a way that the stone-bearing ureter lies obliquely in a comfortable position for the endoknife approaching through the subcostal port (Fig. 10.5(ii)). The endoknife is advanced right up to the stone bulge, but the blade is advanced and locked in the first slot only when one is ready to incise the

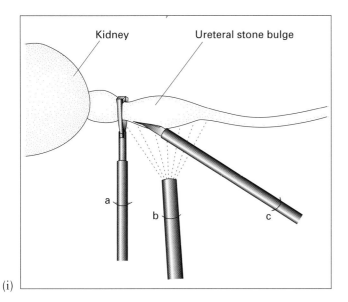

(i)

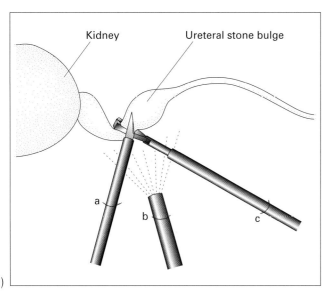

(ii)

Fig. 10.5 (i) The right upper ureter is incised with an endoknife through the iliac port (**c**), while a Babcock through the renal angle port (**a**) steadies the ureter; (ii) A Babcock through the iliac port (**c**) holds the right ureter proximal to the calculus and is depressed against psoas. It is rotated to make the stone-bearing part lie obliquely, so that it can be easily incised through the renal angle port (**a**); **b**, laparoscope port.

ureter. If the angle between the primary and the endoknife ports is very acute, a 30° laparoscope is used to obtain a better view of the blade. The incision is made in an antegrade direction, 1/4 of it being over the dilated ureter and the remaining 3/4 over the stone. The blade is then retracted under vision and the endoknife removed. If the ureteral mucosa has not been divided completely, endoshears are used to complete the incision.

Sometimes it is not possible to hold the proximal ureter if the calculus is very high or if the ureter is grossly dilated or oedematous. If the calculus is high in the ureter, the ureter is pulled down after grasping it distal to the calculus and then incised in an antegrade direction. Retraction of the lower pole of the kidney through the anterior port might be required during this procedure. For a low ureteric calculus, the Babcock holding the ureter just distal to the calculus is pressed against the psoas and rotated in such a way that the ureter becomes S-shaped (Fig. 10.6). The ureter can now even be incised in a retrograde direction, without risk of the calculus migrating proximally, due to the S-curve. If an endoknife is not available, the ureter can be incised with a sharp diathermy electrode, but this is slightly more traumatic. If the stone is lying in a comfortable position, it can be incised through a single accessory port. There is no need to hold it with a Babcock if it has not been dissected circumferentially.

INCISING THE URETER WHEN THE CALCULUS IS IN THE PELVIC URETER

Due to the limited space available in the pelvic retroperitoneum, and a decrease in the angle between the ports caused by a change in the angle of approach, it may be difficult to incise the ureter if it has been grasped proximal to the calculus. It should therefore be grasped below the calculus with a Babcock passed through the iliac port, lifted up and then incised in a retrograde direction with the endoknife inserted through the posterior subcostal port (Fig. 10.7). This necessitates a reversal of the sizes of the two accessory ports to accommodate the 10-mm endoknife. One should resist the temptation to milk the calculus up the ureter, as this might damage the ureter if the calculus is impacted and may sometimes make it difficult to locate the calculus when it is dislodged into the dilated ureter.

REMOVAL AND EXTRACTION OF THE CALCULUS

A gush of urine can be seen as soon as the ureter is incised if the Babcock has been applied distally. Before making an attempt to remove the calculus, one must first ensure that the ureteral mucosa has been completely divided. The calculus is then loosened by freeing it from the ureteral mucosal adhesions with the 5-mm spatula dissector. The calculus can be removed from the ureter by levering it out with the 5-mm dissector

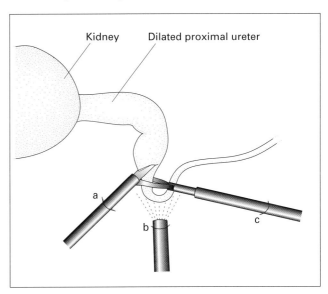

Fig. 10.6 A Babcock through the iliac port (c) holds the ureter distal to the calculus and rotates it to make an S-curve. An endoknife through the renal angle port (a) makes a retrograde incision over the calculus; b, laparoscope port.

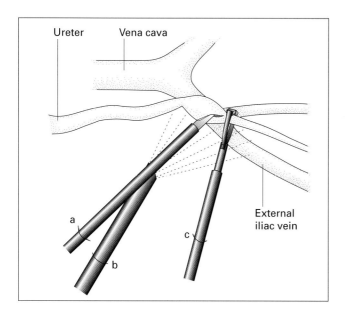

Fig. 10.7 A Babcock through the iliac port (**c**) holds the right pelvic ureter distal to the calculus and lifts it up for the endoknife through the renal angle port (**a**). A 30° laparoscope is used (**b**).

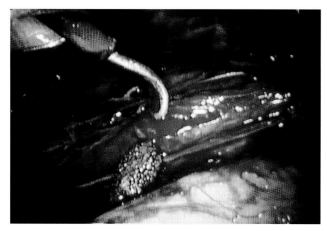

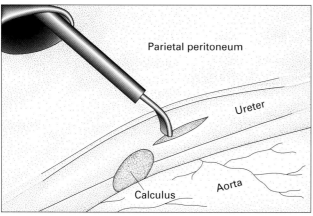

Fig. 10.8 A ureteric calculus has been levered out of the left upper ureter with a 5-mm spatula dissector and is lying over the aorta.

(Fig. 10.8). It can also be removed by pushing it out by angulating the ureter at the level of the incision with the same dissector or preferably with a 7-mm blunt hook. Alternatively, it can be pushed out by angulating the ureter with a Babcock applied just distal to the calculus. If the ureteral incision is rather too small, it should be removed by grasping it with a 5-mm curved grasper.

Ten-millimetre cup forceps are now passed through one of the posterior ports and the calculus is picked up and extracted through the 10-mm port. If it is large, it is removed by pulling it out with the port. The cup forceps have a very strong grip and will allow retrieval of the calculus by stretching the 10-mm track. If the calculus is too large even for this manoeuvre, it is removed either by slightly enlarging the port or by pushing it out through the 2-cm balloon port incision by digital guidance.

FLUSHING OUT RESIDUAL STONES

The ureterotomy site is explored with curved grasping forceps for any residual stones, after re-establishing whatever ports had been removed during the extraction of the calculus. If there is suspicion of a residual stone having migrated up or down the ureter, an attempt can be made to gently squeeze it out with fallopian tube-holding forceps. The ureteral incision is then flushed with normal saline using a 5-mm curved ureteral flushing cannula to wash out any small residual stone fragments. If any more stones are suspected in the proximal dilated ureter or the pelvicalyceal system, they can also be flushed out by inserting a rubber catheter attached to the tip of the ureteral cannula inserted right into the renal pelvis [11]. However, this may not be possible if the ureterotomy incision is below the fourth lumbar vertebra. The Babcock is now placed above the ureteral incision, the rubber catheter attached to the ureteral cannula is inserted into the distal ureter and about 10 ml of normal saline is flushed to ensure its patency. The fluid collecting in the retroperitoneal space is sucked out and any small stones which have been flushed out are removed.

STENTING THE URETER

Stenting of the ureter may be performed to minimize post-operative urinary leak, but in our setting we do not perform it routinely as it almost doubles the total cost to the patient and requires readmission for its removal. If the ureter could not be stented at the start of the procedure due to an impacted calculus, this can be done after removal of the calculus by either pushing up a double-J stent/guide wire assembly or by passing a guide wire through the open-ended catheter placed pre-operatively below the calculus. Alternatively, it could be done intra-operatively, either cystoscopically or retroperitoneoscopically.

SUTURING THE URETER

Meticulous suturing of the ureter is required to minimize post-operative urinary leakage, especially if a stent is not used. Retroperitoneoscopic suturing is difficult compared to the transperitoneal procedure due to space restrictions. The following techniques can be used depending upon the surgeon's skill, experience and resourcefulness.

The standard technique. Using an atraumatic grasper and a needle holder inserted through the two posterior ports the ureteral incision is closed with a continuous or a few interrupted 3/0 or 4/0 catgut sutures and the knots tied intra- or extracorporeally. The procedure can be time-consuming and alternatives in the form of absorbable clips, biocompatible glues and laser welding [12–14] are currently being investigated. Mechanized laparoscopic suturing devices are now also available on the market, which have simplified the procedure.

The clip ligation technique. This is a simple method of closing the ureter without the need for knot tying [11]. A longitudinal mattress suture is inserted with the other end of the suture still lying outside and the needle pulled out through the same port. The ends of the catgut are pulled up and a clip is applied close to the serosa to hold the suture tight. The ends of the catgut are pulled out after cutting it near the clip. Good apposition of the edges, without eversion, is obtained by this method.

The percutaneous technique. The suture is inserted percutaneously over the ureterotomy site by loading it into a 10-cm long needle, but the other end of the suture is not pulled in. After a bite has been taken through the ureteral edges (Fig. 10.9) the knots can be tied extracorporeally after

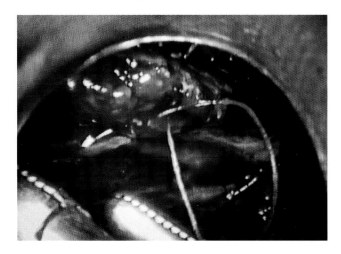

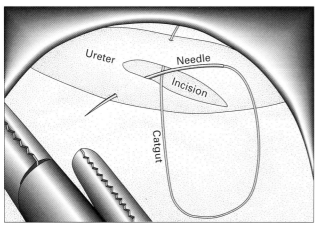

Fig. 10.9 The suture inserted percutaneously has been passed through the cut edges of the ureter.

removing the needle through the same percutaneous track, or intra-corporeally using the twist or the weft and warp technique [15]. The technique is simple as it provides extracorporeal control of the suture and the knots are formed easily around the relatively fixed afferent limb of the suture.

CLOSURE OF PORT SITES

The retroperitoneum is thoroughly checked for blood clots, balloon or stone fragments and bleeding points. If the ureter has not been stented, it should be properly aligned. A tube drain is passed through the iliac or anterior port and its tip positioned by digital or endoscopic guidance. All ports are then removed and the drain connected to a bag after securing it to the skin. The 5-mm ports are closed with a single skin suture, while the others are closed in two or three layers with 2/0 or 3/0 Vicryl. A long-acting local anaesthetic is infiltrated into the skin edges to minimize the post-operative discomfort.

The iliac approach

The anaesthetized patient is placed in a supine position with ipsilateral iliac elevation and the primary port established as described in Chapter 2. The extended iliac technique provides an excellent exposure of the mid-ureter but the lower ureter needs to be dissected endoscopically. The use of a 30° laparoscope is helpful during this dissection.

The balloon dissection of the mid- and part of the lower ureter is sometimes so good that a ureterolithotomy can be performed with a single 10-mm accessory port placed above the iliac crest in the anterior axillary line. However, a second 5-mm accessory port placed just medial to the anterior superior spine, makes the procedure much easier. A third accessory port is rarely required for peritoneal retraction by the second assistant but when necessary is placed above the iliac port.

The surgeon sits on a stool so that he can use the first and the second accessory ports comfortably. The first assistant manipulates the primary port, standing at his side. The ureter can be easily identified arched over the reflected pelvic peritoneum, with the gonadal vessels lying anteriorly and the iliac vessels posteriorly (Fig. 10.10). When it cannot be identified immediately, it should be sought as it crosses the iliac vessels. The rest of the procedure is identical to that performed during a lumbar approach.

Post-operative care

Patients are allowed to take a liquid diet and are mobilized as soon as they have recovered from anaesthesia. The urethral catheter, if present, is removed on completion of the operative procedure. The patient can be discharged with the drain the following day or after it has stopped draining (typically 2–10 days). A combination of trimethoprim and sulphamethoxazole is given until the drain and double-J stent have been removed. Oral analgesics are usually required for 2–3 days post-

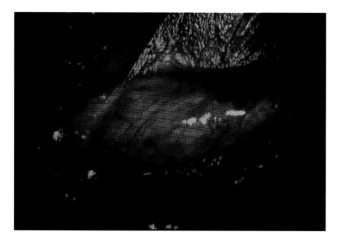

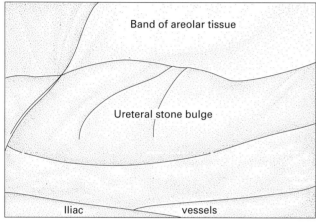

Fig. 10.10 A neatly dissected left lower ureter with the calculus bulge is seen as soon as the laparoscope is inserted after the iliac balloon dissection. A band of areolar tissue is seen above and the iliac vessels below.

operatively. The patients can resume non-strenuous activity after the drain has been removed, and become fully active in 2–4 weeks time.

Results

Although retroperitoneal laparoscopic ureterolithotomy has been performed all over the world, the experience is limited. No complications or failures have been reported in the series of three patients reported by Harewood and colleagues and five by Eden [5,16]. In our series of 30 patients, retroperitoneoscopic ureterolithotomy was successfully performed in 26 cases. The four failures were due to inability to locate the calculus in the ureter in one patient, loss of pneumoretroperitoneum in two patients and dense adhesions in a further patient. They were mostly during the early part of our learning curve and were converted into a mini open procedure by joining two of the incisions along the marked kidney incision line. The calculi were present in the upper ureter in 21 patients, mid-ureter in seven patients and lower ureter in two patients. They were multiple only in one patient and ranged in size from 10 to 40mm in their long axis. The calculi were chronically impacted in all patients and were considered suitable for the procedure as ESWL and endourological procedures were either not available or had failed. One patient had renal failure due to a calculus impacted in the upper ureter in a solitary kidney.

The lumbar approach was used in 24 patients and the iliac approach only in six patients, half of them having an extended procedure. The mini open access technique was used in 24 patients and the closed percutaneous in the remaining six. Three accessory ports were used in 17 patients, mainly during the early part of the practice. However, in 10 patients the procedure could be performed with only two accessory ports and in three with only one accessory port.

The endoknife was used to incise the ureter in 25 patients and electrocautery in five patients. The incisions were much cleaner and more accurate when the endoknife was used. There was excessive prolapse of the ureteral mucosa in one patient due to the drag effect of electrocautery. Most ureterotomies were left open during the early part of the series due to lack of experience and limited availability of operating room time. They were closed only in 10 patients using the standard method in one, clip ligation in three and the percutaneous method in six patients. The ureters were stented 1–2 weeks pre-operatively in two patients for pain control and intra-operatively in four patients. In patients in whom the ureterotomy was left open, urinary leakage stopped within 10 days, except in one case where it continued for a fortnight. All patients were discharged the following day. Urinary drainage stopped in 1–4 days when the ureterotomy was closed and these patients were discharged after the removal of the drain.

The mean operating time was 60 minutes (range 40–150) without ureteral closure and 90 minutes (range 50–140) when the ureter was sutured. There were no major complications in this series. One patient had a peritoneal tear caused by a haemostat during creation of the initial retroperitoneal space, which did not prove to be of any consequence. There was persistence of renal pain in another patient who had had his ureter sutured and who developed ureteral obstruction, which required ureteric stenting two weeks post-operatively. A three-month follow-up intravenous urogram (IVU) showed no abnormality. All patients resumed normal activity within 2–3 weeks.

References

1 Wickham JEA. The surgical treatment of renal lithiasis. In: Wickham JEA, ed. *Urinary Calculus Disease*. New York: Churchill Livingstone, 1979: 145–198.

2 Clayman RV, Preminger GM, Franklin JR, Curry T, Peters PC. Percutaneous ureterolithotomy. *J Urol* 1985; 133: 671–674.

3 Meretyk S, Clayman RV, Myers JA. Retroperitoneoscopy: foreign body retrieval. *J Urol* 1992; 147: 1608–1611.

4 Gaur DD. Laparoscopic operative retroperitoneoscopy: Use of a new device. *J Urol* 1992; 148: 1137–1139.

5 Harewood LM, Webb DR, Pope AJ. Laparoscopic ureterolithotomy: the results of an early series and an evaluation of its role in the management of ureteral calculi. *Br J Urol* 1994; 72: 170–176.

6 Gaur DD. Retroperitoneal laparoscopic ureterolithotomy. *World J Urol* 1993; 11: 175–178.

7 Gaur DD. Retroperitoneal surgery of kidney, ureter and adrenal. *Endosc Surg Allied Technol* 1995; 1: 3–8.

8 Gaur DD. Laparoscopic ureterolithotomy. In: Smith AD, ed. *Controversies in Endourology.* Philadelphia: WB Saunders, 1995: 353–360.

9 Gaur DD. Innovations in Retroperitoneoscopy. Guest lecture at the 7th World Video Urology Congress 1995, Taipei.

10 Low RK, Moran ME. Laparoscopic use of the ureteral illuminator. *Urology* 1993; 42: 455–457.

11 Gaur DD. Retroperitoneal laparoscopy: some technical modifications. *Br J Urol* 1996; 77: 304–306.

12 Eden CG. Alternative techniques for laparoscopic tissue anastomosis in the retroperitoneum. *Endosc Surg Allied Technol* 1995; 1: 29–32.

13 Kram HB, Ocampo HP, Yamaguchi MP, Nathan RC, Shoemaker WC. Fibrin glue in renal and ureteral trauma. *Urology* 1989; 33: 215–218.

14 Neblett CR, Morris JR, Thomsen S. Laser-assisted microsurgical anastomosis. *Neurosurgery* 1986; 19: 914–934.

15 Gaur DD. A simple technique for laparoscopic suturing and knot tying (unpublished observations).

16 Eden CG. Operative retroperitoneoscopy. *Br J Urol* 1995; 76: 125–130.

11 Nephrectomy

J. J. RASSWEILER

The first attempts at endoscopic nephrectomy were made by Coptcoat [1], Wickham and Miller [2], and Weinberg and Smith [3] in the early 1980s and were based on the technique of percutaneous renal stone surgery. The clinical breakthrough, however, was achieved by Clayman and colleagues in 1991 [4] by performing a transperitoneal laparoscopic nephrectomy (TLN). A major criticism of TLN for benign disease, however, is that it requires a transabdominal approach, in contrast to open surgery. As a consequence, both Clayman's [5] and Wickham's [6] groups have since investigated the feasibility of retroperitoneal laparoscopic nephrectomy through experimental and clinical studies. However, their attempts were hampered by their inability to create an effective pneumoretroperitoneum because of the dense areolar tissue binding the fat in the retroperitoneum, which could not be broken down merely by the technique of pneumoinsufflation.

In 1992 Gaur [7] described a pneumatic dissection technique for the retroperitoneum based on balloon insufflation to a maximum pressure of 110 mmHg. He successfully applied this approach for multiple procedures in the retroperitoneum, including simple nephrectomy, renal biopsy, ureterolithotomy and varicocoelectomy [8–10]. Since that time other authors [11,12] have presented their experience using Gaur's technique (Fig. 11.1(a)–(c)) for further indications, such as radical nephrectomy, nephrectomy in children and lumbar sympathectomy, using either pneumatic or hydraulic balloon dissection. In contrast, Mandressi and colleagues have described a technique for the fluoroscopically guided establishment of a pneumoretroperitoneum [13]. We have modified this procedure into a hydraulic endoscopically controlled balloon dissection technique of the retroperitoneal space [12].

Indications

From December 1992 to December 1995 we used this approach to the upper retroperitoneum in 59 patients (Table 11.1) ranging in age from 4 to 82 years.

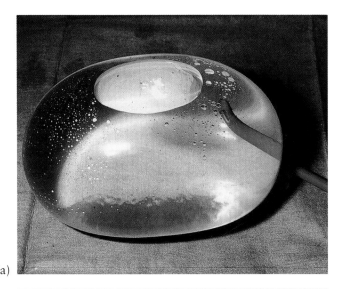

(a)

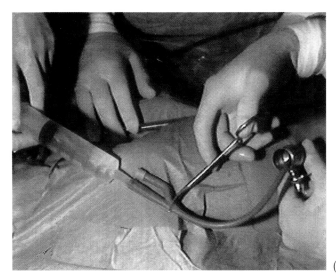

(b)

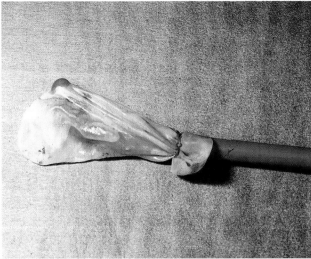

(c)

Fig. 11.1 Hydraulic balloon dissection (Gaur's technique) using a finger of a size 8 surgeon's glove ligated to a red rubber catheter: (a) balloon filled with 300 ml of normal saline; (b) introduction of the catheter via a 10/11-mm trocar sheath and instillation of normal saline using a 60-ml bladder syringe; (c) deflated balloon following use.

Table 11.1 Retroperitoneal laparoscopic nephrectomies performed in the Departments of Urology, Heilbronn and Klinikum Mannheim, from December 1992 to December 1995.

Procedure	Number performed
Retroperitoneal laparoscopic nephrectomy	47
Nephroureterectomy	5
Radical nephrectomy	2
Heminephrectomy	5
Total	59

Simple nephrectomy

This was performed for hydronephrosis, end-stage renovascular disease, chronic pyelonephritis, end-stage stone disease and renal dysplasia (including one 4- and one 14-year-old child). In three cases the patient had had previous abdominal surgery (appendicectomy, cholecystectomy and multiple laparotomies for a retroperitoneal sarcoma) and one patient had had an open pyelolithotomy.

Radical nephrectomy

This was performed for a tumour in a patient with a history of peritonitis; the kidney was removed within Gerota's fascia entirely retroperitone-oscopically.

Nephroureterectomy

This was performed for reflux nephropathy prior to renal transplantation in two cases: one had had previous abdominal surgery, and the other had a primary obstructive megaureter with a non-functioning kidney.

Heminephrectomy

This was performed on duplex systems for removal of either a hydro-nephrotic ($n = 2$) or dysplastic ($n = 3$) moiety.

Patient preparation

The pre-operative preparation is similar to that for patients undergoing open or transperitoneal laparoscopic renal surgery: informed consent, bowel preparation with bisacodyl 10 mg by mouth, cross-matching of blood, peri-operative antibiotics, and prophylaxis against deep vein thrombosis with heparin and elastic stockings.

Access to the retroperitoneum

Under general anaesthesia, the patient is placed in the typical kidney position. No Trendelenburg tilt is necessary. A 15–18-mm incision (Fig. 11.2) is made in the muscle-free triangle between the twelfth rib and the iliac crest, bounded by the lateral edges of the latissimus dorsi and the external oblique muscles. A tunnel down to the retroperitoneal space is created by blunt dissection using Overhold forceps. This tunnel is dilated until an index finger can be introduced to push the peritoneum forwards, thus creating a retroperitoneal cavity for correct placement of the balloon-trocar system (Fig. 11.3).

The balloon-trocar system

The balloon-trocar system consists of the middle finger of a surgeon's glove ligated to an 11-mm metal trocar sheath (Fig. 11.4). Although a purpose-designed disposable balloon trocar exists (Origin Medsystems, Menlo Park, USA; see Fig. 11.4), our experience is that our cheap version

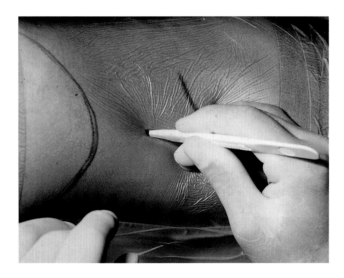

Fig. 11.2 The 15-mm lumbodorsal incision at the muscle-free triangle between the latissimus dorsi and external oblique muscles.

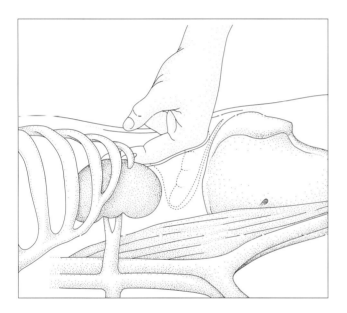

Fig. 11.3 Blunt dissection of the retroperitoneal space with the index finger pushing the peritoneum medially and palpating the psoas muscle and kidney.

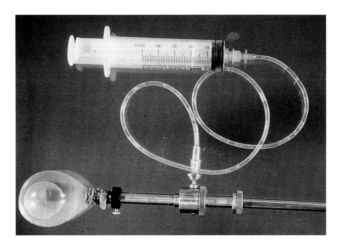

Fig. 11.4 Balloon-trocar system for endoscopically controlled hydraulic dissection of the retroperitoneum. A finger of a surgeon's glove is ligated to the fixation grip of a 12/13-mm metal trocar sheath. The balloon is inflated via the insufflation channel with the telescope inserted to monitor the balloon dissection.

of this system is adequate when used in the manner described below. The 'balloon' of the balloon-trocar system is filled via the insufflation channel of the trocar sheath.

For monitoring the dissecting pressure during inflation the tube which is connected to the insufflation channel of the trocar sheath can be permanently marked at 10-cm intervals. For measurement of the pressure within the balloon, the tube is disconnected from the syringe and held vertically. The column of water in the tube above the kidney should not be allowed to exceed 100 cm (Fig. 11.5).

Hydraulic balloon dissection

Once the latex balloon has been filled with about 50 ml of normal saline the telescope is inserted into the trocar sheath (Fig. 11.6). Once distended,

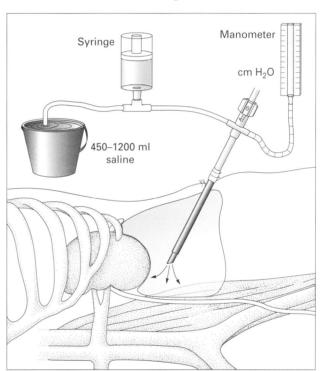

Fig. 11.5 Schematic drawing of endoscopically controlled hydraulic dissection of the retroperitoneum. The intraluminal pressure can be measured manometrically and should not be allowed to exceed 100 cmH$_2$O.

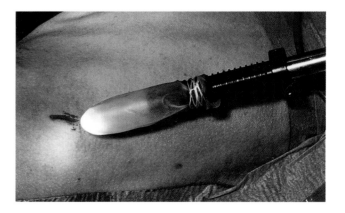

Fig. 11.6 Insertion of the balloon-trocar system.

the balloon becomes transparent and the process of dissection can be monitored under direct vision (Fig. 11.7). It is of great importance that the process of dissection is observed continuously, separating Gerota's fascia from the psoas muscle. If this is not the case, the pressure in the system should be checked manometrically.

The balloon is filled to 400–1000 ml according to the patient's size (children 400–700 ml and adults 700–1000 ml). Although our studies have demonstrated that the maximum capacity of the balloon before rupture is 2000–2400 ml, spontaneous rupture of the balloon may occur earlier, particularly if the intraluminal pressure exceeds 100 cmH$_2$O due to significant adhesions within the retroperitoneum. The balloon is kept fully inflated for 5 minutes to achieve adequate haemostasis within the retroperitoneal space. After desufflation of the balloon, the balloon-trocar system is withdrawn. We then insert a sterile gauze into the retroperitoneal space to keep it dry.

Placement of secondary trocars

Secondary trocars are inserted to one side of an index finger introduced through the primary access wound (Fig. 11.8). To avoid injury to the surgeon's finger a track is first dilated using forceps. Port II (10/11 mm) is manipulated by the surgeon's right hand (scissors and endo-clip applicator) and port III (5 mm) by his left hand (forceps).

The initial wound is closed around the port using a mattress suture to avoid gas leakage. The port is then connected to the CO$_2$ insufflator to establish a pneumoretroperitoneum, with a maximum pressure limit of 15 mmHg and a rate of 3.5 l/min, before retroperitoneoscopy is performed. If necessary, a further 5-mm port (IV) is inserted under endoscopic vision to retract the kidney during dissection. After all the ports have been placed the maximum inflation pressure is reduced to 12 mmHg. As in an open procedure, both surgeon and assistant stand on the dorsal side of the patient.

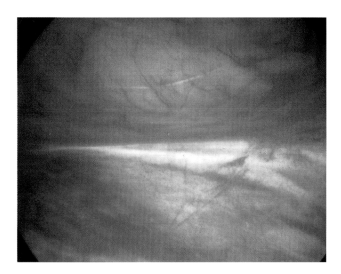

Fig. 11.7 Endoscopic view during balloon dissection. The dense areolar tissue binding the fat in the retroperitoneum is pushed away by the balloon.

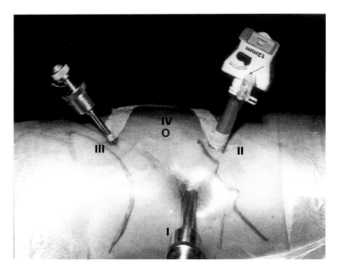

Fig. 11.8 Port placement. The patient is in a standard flank position with the surgeon standing on the dorsal side. Port I (12/13 mm) is for the laparoscope, port II (10/11 mm (or 12 mm for endoGIA)) for the surgeon's right hand, port III (5 mm) for the surgeon's left hand, and port IV (5 mm) for the assistant (IV).

Technique of nephrectomy

Dissection and ligation of the ureter

After incision of Gerota's fascia (Fig. 11.9) the lumbar ureter and gonadal vein can be seen easily in most cases, isolated, double-clipped and transected. In the three cases of nephroureterectomy the lumbar ureter was isolated but not transected at this stage. The upper ureter (Fig. 11.10) serves as a retractor and a guide for proximal dissection towards the hilar vessels.

Dissection of the kidney and securing the renal vessels

In contrast to transperitoneal nephrectomy, the entire kidney is then dissected from Gerota's fascia; it is important that the entire fascia is incised to open up the retroperitoneal space. Attention now turns to dissection of the renal hilum (Fig. 11.11), and here the use of a 30° telescope is very helpful. In most cases the dissection is performed from the ventral aspect. The renal artery and smaller veins are clipped with a 12-mm clip and transected (Fig. 11.12), whereas larger renal veins should be secured with an endoscopic stapler (Endo-GIA 30 (white cartridge); United States Surgical Corporation, Norwalk, Connecticut, USA). For this step the camera has to be transferred to port II to allow insertion of the instrument via port I. Finally, the upper pole of the kidney is dissected. Here one must be aware of the possibility of additional polar arteries. It should be emphasized that the description given above needs to be modified according to each individual pathological and anatomical situation.

Retrieval of the kidney

An organ bag is necessary for entrapment and retrieval of the kidney. One of the best bags for this is the LapSac™ (Cook-Europe), designed by Clayman [14], which is available in different sizes (Fig. 11.13). It is almost

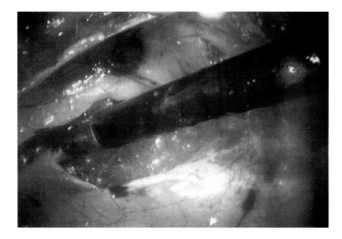

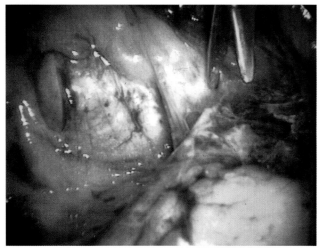

Fig. 11.9 Exposure and incision of Gerota's fascia.

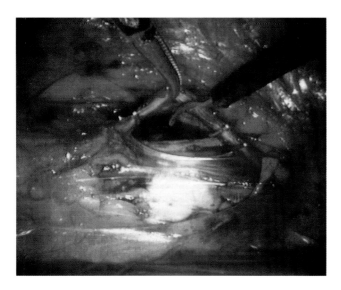

Fig. 11.10 Isolation of the lumbar ureter.

self-expanding inside the abdomen and is very stable, enabling optimal morcellation of the kidney within the bag. One minor disadvantage of the bag is that at least three (and preferably four) ports are necessary to

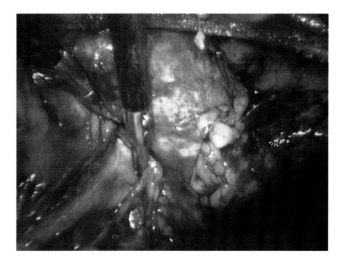

Fig. 11.11 Isolation of the renal pelvis.

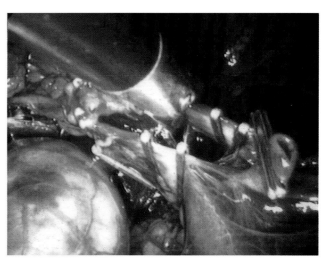

Fig. 11.12 Transection of the renal vein between staples after clipping of the renal artery on the right.

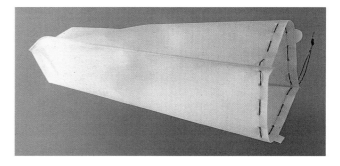

Fig. 11.13 The LapSac™ (Cook-Europe).

entrap the kidney, three to open the LapSac™ and a fourth to place the kidney into the organ bag. Recently, another organ bag with a self-expanding opening has been introduced (Endobag™; Storz, Tuttlingen, Germany), which has proved to be very useful, particularly for the removal of smaller kidneys (Fig. 11.14). It comes folded in an introducer set and has a plastic ring which expands once the bag is released. The kidney can be entrapped within this bag using two or three instruments.

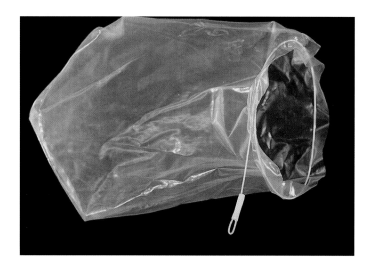

Fig. 11.14 The Endobag™ (Storz, Tuttlingen, Germany).

The material of the Endobag™ is not as stable as that of the LapSac™ but still allows safe morcellation of the organ.

Once the kidney is completely isolated the organ is grasped via port IV and moved caudally, so as not to hinder the introduction of the organ bag. The latter is then held open with one or two graspers and the kidney manoeuvred into the organ bag (Fig. 11.15). After closure of the bag, the 12-mm port is removed and the neck of the bag is then pulled out over the surface of the skin. The port wound is further incised, allowing introduction of the index finger into the organ bag for digital morcellation. Thereafter the fragments are extracted using ring-forceps (Fig. 11.16). The trocar wound should be covered with drapes prior to morcellation to protect it from infection or tumour cells.

After retrieval of the organ bag, the fascia of the external oblique muscle is sutured under vision and the pneumoretroperitoneum re-established to exclude any bleeding. Finally, a drain is inserted via one of the 5-mm ports and all trocar sheaths removed under endoscopic control. The skin over each port wound is then closed intracutaneously.

In the case of nephroureterectomy, after completion of nephrectomy the distal ureter is dissected down to the bladder. If necessary, the lateral umbilical ligament is transected between clips. Since we perform the procedure for benign disease only, we do not remove a cuff of bladder or circumcise the ureteric orifice [15]. For malignant disease, we still prefer a transperitoneal laparoscopic approach in combination with transurethral circumcision of the orifice prior to laparoscopy.

Technique of heminephrectomy

Dissection of the ureter and corresponding vessels

A preliminary retrograde pyelogram and stenting of the respective ureter is mandatory. If the patient is very slim, the stented ureter may be visible through the balloon during retroperitoneal dissection (Fig. 11.17). The ureter is isolated and followed to the hilum where a crossing lower pole

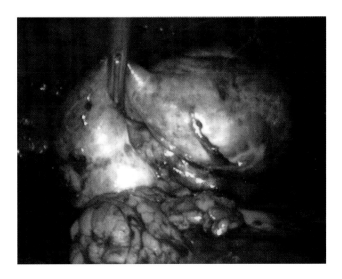

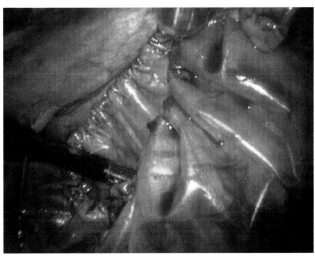

Fig. 11.15 Entrapment of the kidney in the organ bag.

vessel, if encountered (Fig. 11.18), is dissected and clipped. Following this, all arterial and venous branches supplying the lower pole are isolated and transected between endoclips. This results in a purple discoloration of the lower part of the kidney, defining the line of resection.

Division of the parenchyma

Transection of the lower pole of the kidney is commenced with endo-shears and completed with an endoscopic stapler in order to achieve adequate haemostasis. The residual part of the resection plane is then sealed with a new haemostatic patch covered on one side with fibrin glue (Tachocomb™). For adequate haemostasis the patch must be pressed onto the raw surface for 5 minutes (Fig. 11.19). In one patient, we applied two Endoloops (Ethicon, Hamburg, Germany) around the upper pole of the kidney at the line of demarcation. Haemostasis can also be achieved using an argon beam coagulator. The post-operative intravenous pyelogram showed good function of the remaining upper pole (Fig. 11.20).

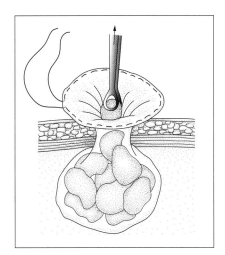

Fig. 11.16 Retrieval of the morcellated kidney using ring forceps.

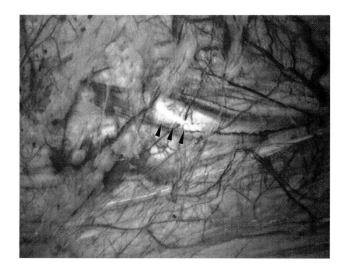

Fig. 11.17 The stented ureter (arrows) is already visible during the endoscopically controlled balloon dissection.

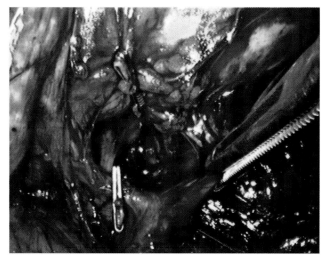

Fig. 11.18 Dissection and clipping of a crossing lower pole segmental artery causing pelviureteric junction obstruction.

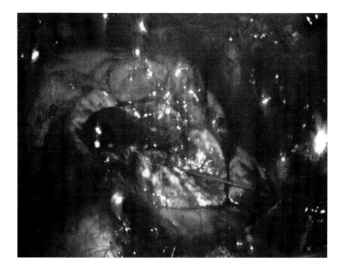

Fig. 11.19 Sealing the resection plane with a haemostatic patch coated with fibrin glue (Tachocomb™).

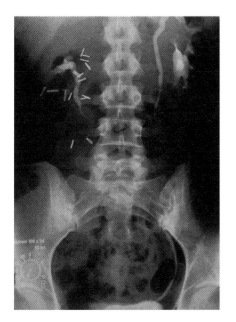

Fig. 11.20 Intravenous pyelogram on the fourth post-operative day demonstrating optimal function of the residual upper part of the right kidney.

Results

The operating times for open, transperitoneal laparoscopic and retroperitoneoscopic nephrectomy by the author are compared in Fig. 11.21. Blood loss was minimal in the great majority of cases.

Complications

Five cases were converted to open nephrectomy. This was due to bleeding in one case, dense perinephric adhesions in two cases and unclear anatomy in two cases.

Complications were noted in five patients: bleeding or haematoma ($n = 3$); subcutaneous abscess ($n = 1$); and pancreatic fistula ($n = 1$). Re-intervention was necessary in two patients, due to bleeding in one and a pancreatic fistula in the second.

Discussion

We feel that the following modifications to Gaur's original description of retroperitoneoscopy have contributed significantly to our excellent results.

Use of the first trocar incision for digital dissection of the retroperitoneal space. The introduction of the index finger to push away the peritoneum, as in open surgery, permits digital localization of the kidney and allows a considerable space to be created prior to introduction of the balloon-trocar system. However, the major advantage of this technique is that the dissection pressure inside the balloon, and hence the risk of balloon rupture, is significantly reduced. The larger trocar incision can also be used later for retrieval and morcellation of the kidney. We now make this extended trocar incision at the beginning, and not as previously reported with transperitoneal laparoscopic nephrectomy [15,16], at the end of the procedure.

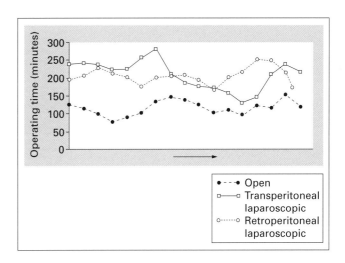

Fig. 11.21 Operating times of consecutive cases of open nephrectomy, transperitoneal laparoscopic nephrectomy and retroperitoneal laparoscopic nephrectomy.

Additionally, this technique of entering the retroperitoneal space has proven to be very safe, easy to perform and reproducible. We feel that it may obviate other approaches for retroperitoneoscopy, i.e. utilizing fluoroscopic-guided placement of the Veress needle [13].

Blunt dissection down only to the psoas muscle and not inside Gerota's fascia. Gaur contends that the operating time is reduced if Gerota's fascia is incised for subfascial placement of the balloon because the whole ureter is dissected by this method. We consider our practice of incision of the fascia overlying the ureter after creation of the pneumoretroperitoneum (Fig. 11.10) to be simple and safer.

Hydraulic balloon dissecting technique. The balloon-trocar system allows the endoscopic observation of balloon dissection, which we feel is one of the major advances in retroperitoneoscopic surgery. We consider that the use of saline for filling the balloon provides better dissecting properties since water is incompressible. However, the position of the balloon must be controlled exactly. In problematic cases (previous surgery or in children) in the past we have serially checked the amount of dissection in the retroperitoneal space by intermittently establishing a pneumoretroperitoneum or by using an ultrasound scanner. However, the current use of preliminary digital dissection allows the extent of dense adhesions to be assessed prior to insertion of the balloon-trocar system. In our experience, severe adhesions, such as after previous renal surgery, cannot be lysed sufficiently by hydraulic balloon dissection and need endoscopic incision.

Monitoring of intraluminal pressure in the balloon-trocar system. To avoid rupture of the latex balloon and possible injury to the peritoneum, it is of major importance to monitor the dissecting pressure in the system and ensure that it is kept $<100\,\text{cmH}_2\text{O}$. Since we use a hydraulic dissecting technique, manometry is quite simple and provides exact data, in contrast to the pneumatic balloon technique proposed by Gaur.

Disadvantages of retroperitoneoscopy

SMALL OPERATIVE FIELD
The use of a 30° telescope can compensate for this, even in children. In difficult cases the most cranial port can be placed in the eleventh intercostal space. However, it must be emphasized that in grossly obese patients, who have a large amount of perirenal fat, the transperitoneal route is preferable.

Advantages of retroperitoneoscopy

SHORTER LEARNING CURVE
One of the major advantages of this new technique is that it uses exactly the same approach to the kidney as open surgery. Thus, in contrast to

Table 11.2 Comparison of transperitoneal laparoscopic nephrectomy (TLN), retroperitoneal laparoscopic nephrectomy (RLN) and open nephrectomy.

	TLN (n = 21)	RLN (n = 23)	Open (n = 19)
Indication			
Hydronephrosis	9	11	11
Chronic pyelonephritis	4	2	5
Renovascular disease	2	4	1
Renal dysplasia	1	2	–
Reflux nephropathy	2	3	1
End-stage nephrolithiasis	3	1	1
Sugical history			
Previous abdominal surgery	1	3	3
Previous retroperitoneal surgery	0	1	1
Results			
Mean operation time (minutes)	202	168	117
Complications	5	1	2
Mean analgesic requirement (vials)	1.8	0.7	3.3
Mean duration of analgesic requirement (days)	2.5	1.0	4.0
Mean post-operative stay (days)	6.9	4.7	10.3

transperitoneal laparoscopic access, the same surgical dissecting principles can be applied: primary isolation of the ureter and dissection of the kidney within Gerota's fascia for simple nephrectomy. As a result, the learning curve is significantly reduced compared with the transperitoneal approach.

REDUCED POST-OPERATIVE MORBIDITY
In accordance with Kerbl and Clayman [17] our initial experience with retroperitoneal laparoscopic nephrectomy (RLN) indicated that this approach results in a further reduction of post-operative morbidity compared with TLN and open surgery (Table 11.2). We therefore currently use a transperitoneal laparoscopic approach only for nephrectomy for malignancy, adrenalectomy and retroperitoneal lymphadenectomy.

SAFETY AND COST
As there is no need for blind puncture with a Veress needle or first trocar, reusable trocars and instruments can be used. With the introduction of endoclip applicators which allow the use of the same clips as in open surgery (Ligaclip extra; Ethicon, Hamburg, Germany) the need for disposable multi-clip applicators has also become questionable. Future use of disposable equipment is likely to be confined to the use of endoscopic staplers for the ligation of large renal veins.

References

1 Coptcoat MJ. Endoscopic tissue liquidisation of the prostate, bladder and kidney. ChM thesis, University of Liverpool, 1990.
2 Wickham JEA, Miller RA. Percutaneous renal access. In: Wickham JEA,

Miller RA, eds. *Percutaneous Renal Surgery*. New York: Churchill Livingstone, 1983: 33–39.

3 Weinberg JJ, Smith AD. Percutaneous resection of the kidney: preliminary report. *J Endourol* 1988; 2: 355–357.

4 Clayman RV, Kavoussi LR, Soper NJ *et al*. Laparoscopic nephrectomy: initial case report. *J Urol* 1991; 146: 278–282.

5 Figenshau RS, Clayman RV, Kavoussi LR, Chandhoke P, Albala DM, Stone AM. Retroperitoneal laparoscopic nephrectomy: laboratory and initial clinical experience. *J Endourol* 1991; 5: S130.

6 Watson GM, Ralph DJ, Timoney AG, Wickham JEA. Laparoscopic nephrectomy: initial experience. *Eur Urol* 1992; 20 (suppl.): 314.

7 Gaur DD. Laparoscopic operative retroperitoneoscopy: use of a new device. *J Urol* 1992; 148: 1137–1139.

8 Gaur DD. Retroperitoneal laparoscopic ureterolithotomy. *World J Urol* 1993; 11: 175–177.

9 Gaur DD, Purohit KC, Agarwal DK, Darshane AS. Laparoscopic ureterolithotomy for impacted lower ureteral calculi: initial case report. *Min Invas Ther* 1993; 2: 267–269.

10 Gaur DD, Agarwal DK, Purohit KC, Darshane AS. Retroperitoneal laparoscopic pyelolithotomy. *J Urol* 1994; 151: 927–929.

11 Janetschek G, Flora G, Biedermann H, Bartsch G. Lumbar sympathectomy by means of retroperitoneoscopy. *Min Invas Ther* 1993; 2: 271–273.

12 Rassweiler JJ, Henkel TO, Stoch C *et al*. Retroperitoneal laparoscopic nephrectomy and other procedures in the upper retroperitoneum using a balloon dissection technique. *Eur Urol* 1994; 25: 229–236.

13 Mandressi A, Buizza C, Antonelli D *et al*. Retro-extraperitoneal laparoscopic approach to excise retroperitoneal organs: kidney and adrenal gland. *Min Invas Ther* 1993; 2: 213–220.

14 Clayman RV, Kavoussi LR, Long SR, Dierks SM, Meretyk S, Soper NJ. Laparoscopic nephrectomy: initial report of pelviscopic organ ablation in the pig. *J Endourol* 1990; 4: 247–251.

15 Rassweiler JJ, Henkel TO, Potempa DM, Coptcoat M, Alken P. The technique of transperitoneal laparoscopic nephrectomy, adrenalectomy and nephroureterectomy. *Eur Urol* 1993; 23: 425–430.

16 Rassweiler J, Henkel TO, Potempa DM *et al*. Transperitoneal laparoscopic nephrectomy: training, technique and results. *J Endourol* 1993; 7: 505–516.

17 Kerbl K, Clayman RV. Advances in laparoscopic renal and ureteral surgery. *Eur Urol* 1994; 25: 1–6.

12 Adrenalectomy

A. MANDRESSI

Historically, the surgical approach to the adrenals has depended on a variety of factors: the size of the gland; the side of the lesion; the patient's habitus; the surgeon's experience; and, most importantly, the pathology affecting the gland. This is because of the preference of some surgeons to perform a regional lymphadenectomy for carcinoma, in addition to an abdominal exploration to exclude the presence of multifocal or ectopic disease when dealing with phaeochromocytoma [1]. These surgeons have favoured a transabdominal approach, which has allowed them to achieve these aims.

Improved pre-operative imaging and radionuclide scanning have now rendered surgical exploration to establish the diagnosis, the site and the multiplicity of satellite or ectopic lesions obsolete. Armed with this information, it is possible to plan the extent of the surgery with some accuracy before putting knife to skin.

Adrenalectomy is traditionally performed through an incision which is disproportionately large compared to the size of the gland, due to its deep position within the retroperitoneum and the extensive dissection necessary to gain surgical access to it. This paradox has stimulated surgeons to investigate a laparoscopic approach for adrenalectomy, not only to reduce the length of the skin incision but also to decrease the tissue dissection involved, in order to reduce operating time, post-operative pain and the morbidity of the procedure. Given that a direct route to the gland is less invasive and more rapid than any other, a retroperitoneal laparoscopic approach to the adrenals would seem the most logical, given their retroperitoneal position. Until recently, it was believed that retroperitoneal laparoscopic adrenalectomy was not feasible [2] due to the abundant and sometimes overwhelming amount of fat surrounding the adrenals, although the use of an ultrasonic surgical system to remove the fat may aid identification of the vessels [3]. In general, only large adrenal masses requiring regional lymphadenectomy are unsuitable for laparoscopic excision.

Pre-operative investigations

Adrenal masses should be assessed to determine whether they are endocrinologically active by measurement of the products of the adrenal cortex and medulla in either the urine or plasma. Computed tomography (CT) should be performed to clearly define both the location and the size of the adrenal gland (Fig. 12.1). Taking into account the tendency of the CT to underestimate the adrenal size, a non-functioning mass larger than 5 cm is an indication for surgery, because the probability of finding cancerous cells within it increases as the volume increases. A diagnostic problem arises when the non-functioning solid mass is smaller than 5 cm. In this case, magnetic resonance imaging (MRI) might be of use as a lesion with a high signal intensity in T2 weighted images is likely to be a carcinoma [4]. When the T2 image is equivocal, follow-up MRI scanning is advisable to monitor gland growth. A further aid to diagnosis is offered by fine needle aspiration cytology.

For cystic masses, regardless of size, the diagnostic alternatives lie between MRI and cyst puncture. An adrenal cyst should be removed if the cyst aspirate is not clear or a mass persists following aspiration. In patients with suspected phaeochromocytoma both CT and MRI scans should be performed, in addition to [131I]metaiodobenzylguanidine radionuclide scanning, to localize the lesion and to rule out the presence of multifocal lesions. A plain abdominal X-ray should be performed to obtain information on the position of the kidney with respect to the overlying ribs and pleural cavity.

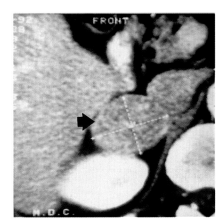

Fig. 12.1 Computed tomogram of a right phaeochromocytoma (arrow).

Indications

The indications for laparoscopic adrenal surgery are the same as for open surgery. Laparoscopic adrenal surgery began in the early 1990s [2,5–10] following the rise in popularity of a laparoscopic approach to peritoneal and retroperitoneal organs [11]. Although initially reserved for small masses, the indications were soon widened (Table 12.1) and included excision of phaeochromocytomas and larger masses [12]. However, the size of the gland still seems to be a limit for laparoscopic surgery: to date the maximum diameter of the gland removed by either a transabdominal or retroperitoneal laparoscopic approach has not exceeded 6 cm. Adrenal malignancies should not be removed by laparoscopy.

Preparation of the patient

Informed consent is obtained from the patient. Lung function should be optimized pre-operatively in patients with airways disease, as this will inevitably be compromised intra-operatively by the patient's prone position.

The patient is prepared for surgery in a routine fashion and is shaved from the thorax to the groin. No preliminary bowel preparation is needed with the extraperitoneal approach. We routinely use short-term paren-

Functioning and non-functioning adenomas
Hyperplastic glands in Conn's sydrome
Phaeochromocytomas
Adrenal cysts yielding an unclear aspirate

Table 12.1 Suitable indications for laparoscopic adrenalectomy.

teral antibiotic prophylaxis with a broad-spectrum agent. Following induction of anaesthesia, two venous cannulae, a nasogastric tube and a urinary catheter are placed.

Per-operative anaesthetic monitoring consists of continuous ECG, measurement of end-tidal carbon dioxide (CO_2) and pulse oximetry. Pulmonary static compliance and both mean and peak airway pressures should be monitored as well. Central venous and arterial lines should be inserted in patients undergoing surgery for phaeochromocytoma, who are at risk of heart failure. Blood pressure control in these patients during the operation is achieved either with an alpha-blocker, such as phentolamine, or with nitroprusside.

Patient positioning

In our initial report [8] of the use of direct CO_2 insufflation for nephrectomy and adrenalectomy, the procedures were performed with patients in the prone position. With increased experience it became apparent that, for nephrectomy, the procedure was technically easier with the patient in the flank position. However, the prone position appeared to be superior for adrenalectomy [13].

The patient is cystoscoped in the lithotomy position and a ureteral catheter placed in the renal pelvis ipsilateral to the gland being removed. The patient is then turned prone, with the arms extended above the head. Foam supports are placed under the thorax and under the hips to allow free expansion of the abdomen (Fig. 12.2) and better expansion of the retroperitoneum. It is worth stressing the importance of sufficient elevation of the hips and thorax, since the adequacy of the retroperitoneal workspace depends on this. The patient's skin is then prepared and draped with a sterile disposable adhesive sheet in routine fashion.

Creation of the retroperitoneal space

The kidney and ureter are visualized by fluoroscopy. In obese patients, injection of contrast may be necessary to identify these structures. The Veress needle is then inserted exactly halfway between the medial aspect

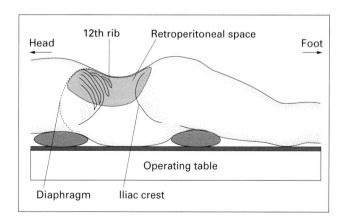

Fig. 12.2 Patient positioning.

of the lower pole of the kidney and the ureter. The Veress needle is gently angulated medially and the corresponding movement of the ureter confirmed fluoroscopically to ensure the correct location of the needle.

Insufflation of the retroperitoneum with CO_2 at 2 l/min is then commenced until 0.5 litre has been insufflated. Manipulation of the needle may be necessary if the maximum pre-set pressure limit of 18 mmHg is temporarily exceeded. The space created by CO_2 insufflation is visualized by fluoroscopy (Fig. 12.3): a crescent of radiolucency should outline the lower pole of the kidney and the ureter. If there is sufficient space for the insertion of the first trocar insufflation can now be stopped, otherwise it should be continued until 1 litre of CO_2 has been insufflated.

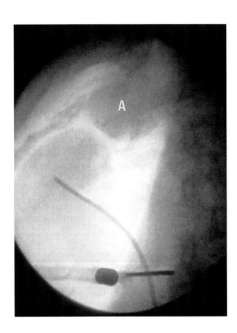

Fig. 12.3 Fluoroscopy demonstrating a lucent area in the left (the patient is prone) retroperitoneal space created by direct insufflation of CO_2. The ureteral catheter is in view. A, left adrenal adenoma.

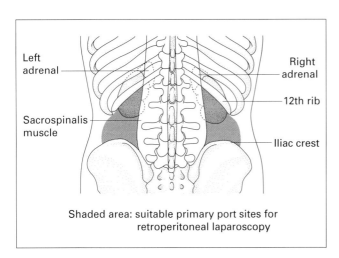

Shaded area: suitable primary port sites for retroperitoneal laparoscopy

Fig. 12.4 Relationship of the twelfth rib, sacrospinalis muscle, kidney and adrenal gland, as viewed from the back.

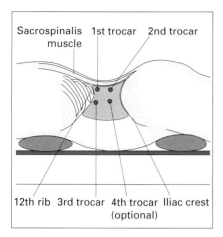

Fig. 12.5 Port placement for left retroperitoneoscopic adrenalectomy. The patient is prone and is viewed from the left.

Placement of trocars

We prefer to use disposable trocars, as they are lighter and less bulky than reusable ones. Moreover, with a disposable trocar, because of its plastic body, there is no risk of discharging stored current when the electro-cautery is in use. The first trocar is inserted at the posterior angle between the twelfth rib and the sacrospinalis muscle (Fig. 12.4) when fluoroscopy shows a lucent area wide enough to outline the renal lower pole. The skin is incised over 1 cm to allow free passage of the 10/11-mm trocar. The insufflation tubing is connected to the trocar and the Veress needle is removed. A 10-mm 0° laparoscope is inserted and the endoscopic view compared with the fluoroscopic image for orientation. Two further trocars are then inserted approximately 3 cm apart (Fig. 12.5); a further port may be useful to avoid the time-consuming exchange of instruments when irrigation and aspiration are needed. The depth of port insertion is controlled fluoroscopically by introducing forceps to determine the depth of the sheath and the position of the instruments in the operative field: these images should be compared with the endoscopic view. The ports are fixed to the skin with nylon sutures.

The laparoscope is inserted into the lower medial port, and the dissector and the scissors are placed in the upper lateral and upper medial ports, respectively. One port is left free for the suction/irrigation probe, if needed. Unless left-handed, the surgeon stands on the side of the adrenalectomy, with the assistant on the opposite side. Two monitors are preferable to allow each surgeon to view the operation comfortably.

Dissection

The perinephric fat on the posteromedial aspect of the kidney is diathermied, cut and detached from the renal capsule, creating a path to the adrenal from the lower to the upper pole (Fig. 12.6). At the upper pole, the kidney should be freed from the fat that is adherent to the adrenal (Fig. 12.7).

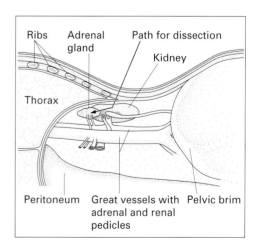

Fig. 12.6 Path of dissection for left retroperitoneoscopic adrenalectomy.

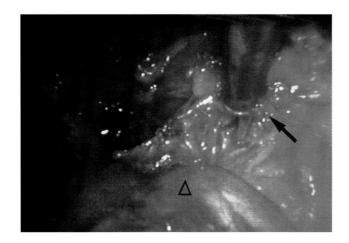

Fig. 12.7 The upper pole of the kidney (Δ) has been dissected from the adrenal (arrow), to which the fat remains adherent.

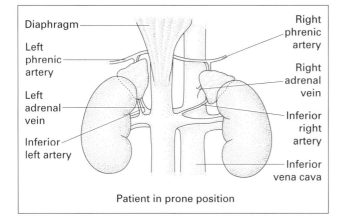

Fig. 12.8 Arterial inflow and venous drainage of the adrenal glands.

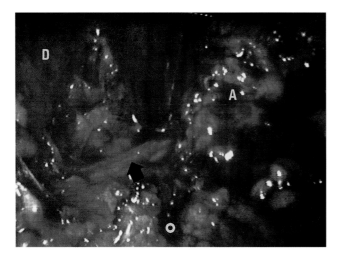

Fig. 12.9 Inferior right adrenal vascular pedicle (arrow). D, diaphragm; A, adrenal; o, IVC covered with fat.

Right adrenalectomy

The dissection of the upper pole advances anteriorly towards the hilar fat, where particular attention should be paid to identify the inferior arterial supply of the adrenal (Figs 12.8 and 12.9), as it passes from medial to lateral between the upper pole of the kidney and the adrenal, branching before reaching the gland. Having carefully dissected away the surrounding fat, the inferior artery is occluded proximally with two clips and distally with one, and subsequently divided. By dissecting the fat just below the divided artery, the inferior vena cava (IVC) appears as a ribbon lying anteromedial to the kidney and disappearing into the fat beneath the adrenal. Following the IVC upwards and clearing the fat from its posterior aspect, brings into view the adrenal vein, which appears as a straight connection between the vena cava and the gland (Fig. 12.10): three clips are placed proximally and one distally before the vein is cut. The anterior dissection of the gland is then completed (Fig. 12.11). Retracting the adrenal laterally once it has been dissected off the diaphragm reveals the superior arterial supply, which is clipped and cut. This leaves only the posterior and lateral aspects of the gland still attached by fat, which is diathermied and divided whilst applying medial and inferior retraction.

Left adrenalectomy

The dissection of the upper pole of the kidney is continued towards the anteromedial hilar fat, where the inferior arterial supply is identified as it

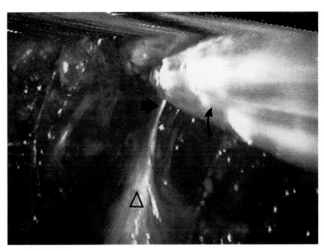

Fig. 12.10 Right adrenalectomy. The short arrow indicates the short right vein being clipped. The curved arrow shows the movement of the stapler as it lifts the gland whilst stapling the vein. Δ, IVC.

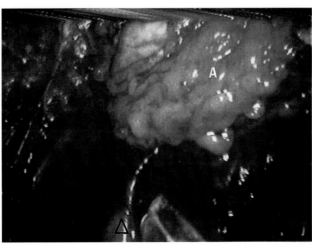

Fig. 12.11 The adrenal (A) covered by its fat is still adherent to the roof of the workspace. The inferior vena cava (Δ) has been dissected from adjacent fat and the right adrenal vein (arrow) has been clipped.

passes laterally directly from the aorta to branch in the gland. The inferior artery is secured proximally with two clips and distally with one and then cut. It is worth emphasizing that at this stage no adrenal dissection has yet been performed. Dissection of the hilar fat reveals the left adrenal vein emerging perpendicularly from the renal vein. It is clipped proximal to the origin of the renal vein and divided. Once the vein is secured the dissection can proceed apace, detaching the gland from the diaphragm and reaching the upper posteromedial aspect of the gland to identify the upper vascular pedicle (Fig. 12.12), where both the superior arterial supply and the phrenic vein should be clipped and cut. The anterior and lateral aspects of the gland can then easily be freed by following Gerota's fascia, completing the dissection and mobilization of the gland.

Removal of the gland

An 'Endo-pouch™', rolled into a 10-mm tube and mounted on an introducer, is introduced into the retroperitoneal space through one of the two medial ports leaving only the string outside. The mouth of the bag is

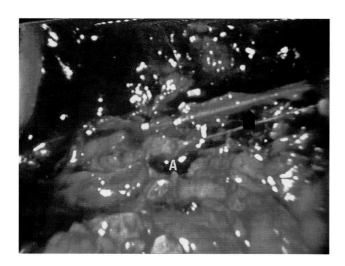

Fig. 12.12 Superior artery (arrow) of the left adrenal gland (A).

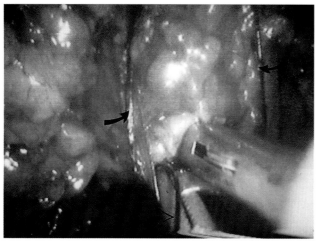

Fig. 12.13 The adrenal is placed into the Endo-pouch™. The two curved arrows indicate the drawstring. The open arrow indicates the string emerging from the port. Note that whilst one pair of forceps holds the bag, the other pushes in the gland.

opened with grasping forceps and the adrenal placed within it (Fig. 12.13). The port is then removed and bag delivered by pulling on the string. The skin incision may need to be enlarged, depending on the size of the specimen. This manoeuvre is viewed endoscopically to ensure the integrity of the bag.

A suction drain is inserted through a port and positioned under endoscopic control. The 1-cm port sites are closed with nylon sutures and the wound through which the gland was delivered is closed in two layers with polyglycolic acid and nylon sutures.

Results

The patient demographics and results of the author's series are summarized in Table 12.2. A single procedure (excision of right phaeochromocytoma) was converted to an open operation at a late stage after insertion of an additional port through the pleura, causing a pneumothorax. Adrenalectomy was completed via an open loin approach. The mean operating time of the successfully operated cases was 2 hours and 50 minutes. The maximum blood loss during the retroperitoneoscopic procedures was 100 ml. Subcutaneous light emphysema due to CO_2 absorption was observed in one case and spontaneously resolved within a few hours.

All patients had their catheters removed and commenced an oral diet on the first post-operative day. All patients had a chest X-ray on the first post-operative day, all of which were normal. No patient required major analgesics. The mean post-operative hospitalization was 4.8 days.

Discussion

Feasibility

Our experience of extraperitoneal (Table 12.2) and transperitoneal laparoscopy suggests that direct CO_2 insufflation with the patient in the modified prone position allows a direct and rapid means of creating a retroperitoneal space large enough for adrenal dissection. The operative

Table 12.2 Patient demographics and results of the author's series.

Patient number	Age	Diagnosis	Side	Size (cm)	Operating time (minutes)	Blood loss (ml)	Discharge (post-operative day)
1	57	Phaeochromocytoma	R	3.5 x 2 x 1	210	<100	4
2	24	Cyst	R	5 x 3 x 0.5	150	<100	4
3	42	Adenoma	L	4 x 3 x 2	170	<100	5
4	39	Cushing's syndrome	R	3.5 x 3 x 2	165	<100	7
5	54	Cushing's sydrome	L	2 x 1.5 x 1.2	160	<100	5
6	25	Phaeochromocytoma	R	6 x 5 x 4.5	Open surgery	350	8
7	56	Conn's syndrome	R	2 x 1.5 x 1.2	150	<100	4
8	59	Phaeochromocytoma	R	4 x 2.5 x 3	150	<100	4
9	47	Phaeochromocytoma	R	4 x 2.5 x 3	150	<100	6

strategy outlined above ensures that the adrenals are easily located, without recourse to the use of additional detecting devices, as described in other transabdominal experiences [14].

Safety

A minimal access approach to adrenalectomy additionally offers an opportunity to minimize the manipulation of the gland being removed for phaeochromocytoma before the occlusion of venous drainage, thereby limiting the risks to the patient caused by large swings in intra-operative blood pressure.

With the patient in the prone position, the sacrospinalis muscle protects the IVC and aorta from injury during insertion of the first trocar. In our series, there were no vascular injuries, neither was the peritoneum opened in any case. The modified prone position also allows free expansion of the retroperitoneal space and thereby reduces IVC compression against the spine, in contrast with conventional pneumoperitoneum.

Effectiveness

All patients reported feeling well and those operated on for hypertension had a normalization of their blood pressure. Sonography did not demonstrate any structural abnormalities. All patients underwent a repeat examination two months following surgery, when nothing abnormal was detected.

Invasiveness

A major criticism of laparoscopic urological procedures until recently was that they required a transperitoneal approach as no organ of interest for the urologist is located within the peritoneal cavity. Retroperitoneoscopic urological surgery avoids peritoneal violation and thereby most of the complications associated with classic laparoscopy, such as bowel injury, trauma to epigastric vessels and errors during peritoneal insufflation (such as preperitoneal insufflation and pneumo-omentum). The need for extensive colonic mobilization and liver and spleen retraction are avoided, reducing the risk of paralytic ileus. Peritoneal adhesions, which represent a relative contraindication to transperitoneal laparoscopy pose no hazards during retroperitoneoscopy.

Table 12.3 Cost comparison of retroperitoneoscopic and open adrenalectomy.

Item	Retroperitoneoscopy ($US)	Open surgery ($US)
Materials	4 800	650
Operating room	3 200	3 200
Hospitalization	3 200	6 400
Medications	160	360
Total	**11 360**	**10 610**

Cost

The economic advantage of retroperitoneoscopic adrenalectomy is demonstrated in Table 12.3. Although the absolute costs involved will vary between institutions, the ratios will remain roughly constant.

Conclusions

A retroperitoneoscopic approach to the retroperitoneal organs is a feasible method, with all the advantages of minimally invasive surgery and without the complications of transperitoneal laparoscopy. The deep location of the adrenal glands within the retroperitoneum suggests that the retroperitoneal laparoscopic approach in prone position is the best option, as it avoids peritoneal violation and a large surgical incision.

References

1 Libertino JA, Novick JE. Adrenal surgery. *Urol Clin North Am* 1989; 16: 417–606.
2 Gagner M, Lacroix A, Prinz RA *et al.* Early experience with laparoscopic approach for adrenalectomy. *Surgery* 1993; 114: 1120–1125.
3 Suzuki K, Fujita K, Ushiyama T, Mugiya S, Kageyama S, Ishikawa A. Efficacy of an ultrasonic surgical system for laparoscopic adrenalectomy. *J Urol* 1995; 154: 484–486.
4 Reinig JW, Doppelman JL, Dwyer AJ, Johnson AR, Knop RH. Adrenal masses differentiated by MR. *Radiology* 1986; 158: 81–89.
5 Higashihara E, Tanaka Y, Horie S *et al.* Laparoscopic adrenalectomy: the initial three cases. *J Urol* 1993; 149: 973–976.
6 Fernandez-Cruz L, Benarroch G, Torres E, Astudillo E, Saenz A, Taura P. Laparoscopic approach to the adrenal tumors. *J Laparoendosc Surg* 1993; 3: 541–546.
7 Suzuki K, Kageyama S, Ueda D *et al.* Laparoscopic adrenalectomy: clinical experience with 12 cases. *J Urol* 1993; 150: 1099–1102.
8 Mandressi A, Buizza C, Antonelli D *et al.* Extraperitoneal laparoscopic approach to excise retroperitoneal organs: kidney and adrenal gland. *Min Invas Ther* 1993; 2: 213–220.
9 Rassweiler JJ, Henkel TO, Potempa DM, Coptcoat M, Alken P. The technique of transperitoneal laparoscopic nephrectomy, adrenalectomy and nephroureterectomy. *Eur Urol* 1993; 23: 425–430.
10 Go H, Takeda M, Takahashi H *et al.* Laparoscopic adrenalectomy for primary aldosteronism: a new operative method. *J Laparoendosc Surg* 1993; 3: 455–459.
11 Clayman RV, Kavoussi LR, Soper NJ, Albala DM, Figenshau RS, Chandhoke PS. Laparoscopic nephrectomy: review of the initial ten cases. *J Endourol* 1992; 2: 127–132.
12 Gill IS, Clayman RV, McDougall EM. Advances in urological laparoscopy. *J Urol* 1995; 154: 1275–1294.
13 Mandressi A, Buizza C, Antonelli D, Chisena S, Servadio G. Retroperitoneoscopy. *Ann Urol* 1995; 29: 91–96.
14 Guazzoni G, Montorsi F, Bergamaschi F *et al.* Effectiveness and safety of laparoscopic adrenalectomy. *J Urol* 1994; 152: 1375–1378.

13 Tissue approximation techniques

C. G. EDEN

The history of surgery shows that it has evolved through three discrete phases: surgery for diagnosis, surgical ablation of diseased organs and, lastly, reconstructive surgery. Laparoscopy has only recently entered the third and final phase of its evolution, as evidenced by the small but steadily increasing number of reports of reconstructive laparoscopy in the scientific literature. It is apparent from most of these efforts that the operating times are long, and that the majority of this time is taken up by tissue reconstruction. The reason for this is well known to those surgeons who have attempted reconstructive laparoscopy: endoscopic suturing is difficult. The recent development of a semi-automated suturing device (Fig. 13.1), which passes a needle from one jaw, through the tissues

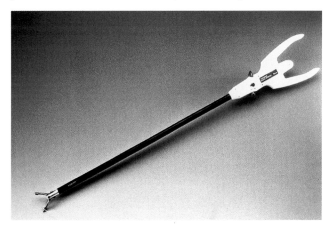

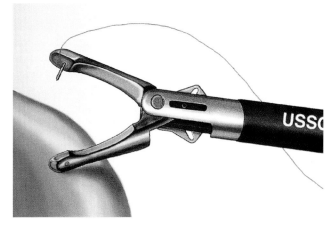

Fig. 13.1 The Endo Stitch™ semi-automated suturing device (USSC, Norwalk, Connecticut, USA).

within the jaw, to the other goes some way towards addressing this problem, but in its present form it is unsuitable for the accurate apposition of fine structures, such as the ureter. Additionally, the suture holes made by this instrument are unnecessarily large, since the needle is available only in one size and the suture material is swaged to its middle, rather than to its end.

Not only is laparoscopic suturing difficult for the ergonomic reasons stated in Table 13.1, but it may also not be the best method of tissue approximation anyway, since (i) when a suture loop is pulled tight, the tissue within its concavity is rendered ischaemic, and (ii) suturing is incapable of producing an anastomosis which is immediately watertight (except in the vascular tree, due to the rapid deposition of fibrin), by virtue of the suture holes at the anastomosis. This may be of great potential importance in the biliary tree and renal tract, since bile and urine are intensely irritant to tissues and since the inflammatory reaction provoked by the extravasation of these fluids may prejudice the long-term patency of the anastomosis by provoking local fibrosis, which may lead to a stricture. What then are the alternatives?

Staples and clips

Staples, such as in linear (Fig. 13.2) and circular (Fig. 13.3) stapler-cutters, are eminently suitable for intestinal side-to-side and end-to-end anastomosis, respectively, but are clearly unsuited to any task which is more delicate, or which involves the biliary tree or the urinary tract, due to the lithogenicity of the titanium staples. End-closure titanium clips, such as those used in laparoscopic herniorrhaphy, have been used by Schuessler to reposition a mobilized colonic flexure over a reconstructed pelviureteric junction, but are large and also lithogenic and therefore unsuited to bile duct or ureteric closure. An absorbable clip has recently been developed by the United States Surgical Corporation, but the deformation characteristics of Polysorb™ (USSC, Norwalk, Connecticut, USA) necessitate the production of a clip which is too large for endoscopic application, let alone the apposition of fine structures.

Tissue adhesives

A number of adhesive systems have been investigated since the 1960s: rubber lattices; nylon systems; epoxy resins; vinyl-containing polymers; polyvinyl alcohol; polyvinylamine, polyvinylpyrrolidone; polyethyleneimine; phosphonyl chloride-terminated polyols; anhydrides; polyacrylates; isocyanates; rapidly polymerizing monomers; formaldehyde resins; and

Two-dimensional image (usually)
Long instruments, which exaggerate tremor
Instruments capable of pivoting only about a single fulcrum
Confined workspace

Table 13.1 Difficulties with laparoscopic suturing.

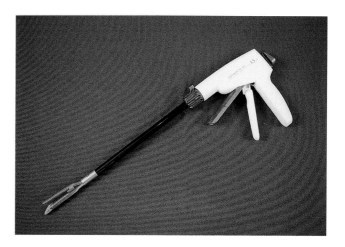

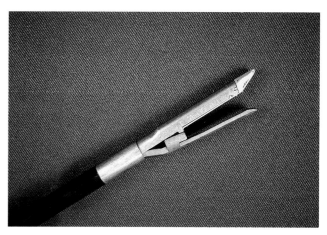

Fig. 13.2 A 35-mm linear stapler-cutter (Ethicon EndoSurgery, Edinburgh, UK).

fibrinogen. Of these, only the latter three have shown sufficient promise to warrant evaluation *in vivo*.

Cyanoacrylates

The alkyl cyanoacrylates were the earliest group of adhesive compounds to attract widespread interest and evaluation. Contact with water causes anionic polymerization of the monomer in an exothermic reaction and tissue adhesion is achieved through two independent mechanisms: molecular attraction (specific adhesion) and interlocking of the polymerized form on irregular surfaces (mechanical adhesion).

However, the application of cyanoacrylates to tissues is also followed by an inflammatory reaction, the magnitude of which is inversely proportional to the length of the monomer chain. The methyl ester has been found to cause medial necrosis in glued canine carotid and femoral arterial anastomoses [1]. This necrosis may lead to fusiform aneurysms at the site of the glued anastomosis and thrombotic occlusion of arteries smaller than 2mm in diameter. It has also been implicated in the fatal rupture of an intracranial aneurysm which was coated with methyl

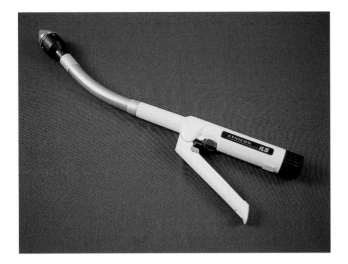

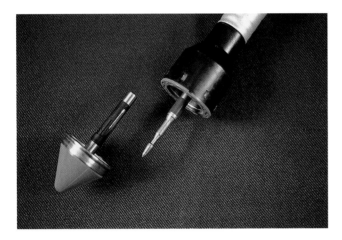

Fig. 13.3 A 33-mm circular stapler-cutter (Ethicon EndoSurgery, Edinburgh, UK).

cyanoacrylate in an attempt to reinforce its thin wall. Methyl cyano-acrylate appears to inhibit the ingrowth of granulation tissue into subcu-taneously implanted Ivalon sponges, but with no apparent long-term deleterious effects. Additionally, there is evidence of direct neurotoxicity of the methyl homologue in both the central and peripheral nervous systems [2]. These effects may be mediated through the production of for-maldehyde during hydrolytic degradation of the methyl polymer. Finally, methyl-2-cyanoacrylate has been shown to be lithogenic in urine.

N-butyl-2-cyanoacrylate (Davis & Geck, Gosport, UK) is the only currently available cyanoacrylate and is licensed for closure of minor skin wounds. For the reasons stated above it is not licensed for internal use.

Gelatin resorcins

The combination of gelatin, resorcin and formaldehyde in appropriate proportions produces a polymer which has a short hardening time, no inherent toxicity and which is absorbed within 2–3 months. However, care must be taken to avoid the addition of an excessive amount of formaldehyde, which is histotoxic. A gelatin resorcin preparation is currently commercially available with 35% formaldehyde and is marketed as 'GRF biological glue' (Laboratoires EHS, Paris, France).

A study of the use of gelatin resorcin glue for the repair of experimentally produced injuries in a canine model showed that the immediate strength of the repair was sufficient to withstand right ventricular pressure. Resection of the various glued tissues at 6 months demonstrated less inflammatory reaction than that seen after tissue repair using cyanoacrylates [3]. Gelatin resorcin glue has also been used successfully to appose the inner and outer arterial layers in the repair of human aortic dissection, both with and without reinforcing sutures with excellent long-term results.

Fibrin glue

The exposure of fibrinogen to calcium and thrombin results in its conversion to a fibrin monomer, which in turn is converted to a stable cross-linked polymer (Fig.13.4). An adhesive bond is formed within a few seconds by the covalent bonding of fibrin and collagen, gaining the majority of its maximum tensile strength within 3–5 minutes. The polymerization reaction generates no heat and the fibrin glue provokes minimal local inflammatory reaction [4]. *In-vitro* experiments suggest that the stabilized fibrin structure may stimulate fibroblasts to grow and promote healing [5]. Ultimately, the fibrin is completely removed by fibrinolysis.

Tisseel™ (Immuno AG, Vienna, Austria) is the most widely available commercially manufactured fibrin glue and is made from highly concentrated fibrinogen and clotting factors from pooled human blood. Its two components are heat-treated fibrinogen in bovine-derived aprotinin (an inhibitor of fibrinolysis) and human thrombin in calcium chloride; these require preliminary reconstitution and warming to 37°C before loading into two separate syringes for synchronous application through a common needle. Alternatively, the glue may be applied using a specially

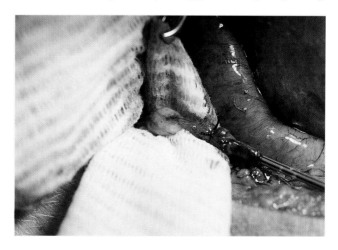

Fig. 13.4 Experimental fibrin-glued ureteric anastomosis.

designed atomizer. Although available in Europe on a 'named patient only' basis, Federal Drug Administration guidelines prohibit the use of pooled human blood products in the USA for fear of transmission of hepatitis and the human immunodeficiency virus. Although there have been no reports of viral transmission through fibrin glue, the concern about this possibility has led to interest in the preparation of fibrin glue from autologous blood [6]. The residual worry regarding the human source of thrombin and bovine source of aprotinin is likely to be overcome in the future by the use of recombinant DNA technology for their production.

Since fibrin glue simulates the final phases of normal blood coagulation it is not surprising that it has also been used successfully as a haemostat in a variety of clinical situations, including following splenic, hepatic, renal and ureteric trauma, and bleeding from nephrostomy tracts after percutaneous nephrolithotomy.

Fibrin and fibrinogen have been used in surgery for tissue approximation and haemostasis since 1940, when Young and Medawar attempted to anastomose nerves. The immediate bond strength of fibrin glue was thought, until recently, to be poor and most investigators consequently employed tension sutures to protect the glue line from the immediate disruptive forces, such as during anastomosis of canine common bile duct [7] and closure of rat cystotomy [8]. This practice makes comparison of anastomotic leak rate, patency and strength with that of sutured anastomoses difficult since glued anastomoses may fare better simply due to the insertion of fewer sutures, with the consequent production of less ischaemia and inflammation. A study avoiding the use of stay sutures entirely has been reported by Niederberger. His group studied sutureless vasovasostomy in a rabbit model, using fibrin glue from a single human source [9]. At 4 weeks, comparison of the glued anastomoses with microsurgically sutured controls demonstrated a similar patency rate (80%) and significantly greater tensile strength in the glued group, in which there was also no sperm granuloma formation. In Ball's comparative study of 10/0 nylon sutures, fibrin glue and CO_2 laser welding for rat vasovasostomy, fibrin glue proved to be superior to both of the other modalities in terms of higher patency (89%) and pregnancy (85%) rates, as well as the lowest granuloma rate (18%) and the shortest operating time [10].

A recent comparative study of the use of fibrin glue to augment high-risk colonic closure in a rat model demonstrated an inferior clinical and radiological outcome in the glue-augmented group, compared with non-glued controls [11]. There was also a higher incidence of perianastomotic adhesions. The authors suggest that the unfavourable outcome in this group may have been due to the production of a stable fibrin polymer by aprotinin, which resisted invasion by vascular granulation tissue and so impaired healing. The higher incidence of perianastomotic adhesions may also have been attributable to the use of aprotinin, as reported in other studies [12,13]. Additionally, high concentrations of fibrinogen and thrombin have been shown to adversely affect neutrophil and macrophage activity and so impair wound healing [13]. Results from a recent animal study [14] suggest that the formulation of commercially available fibrin adhesive is not optimal for tissue approximation, and demonstrated that fibrin glue with a fibrinogen concentration of approximately 39 g/l and a thrombin concentration of 200–600 units/ml with no added factor XIII resulted in the best wound stress, energy absorption and elasticity values.

McKay and colleagues have performed the only published study investigating the laparoscopic use of fibrin glue for reconstruction [15]: they confirmed the feasibility of laparoscopic porcine ureteric reanastomosis, but unfortunately further conclusions from this study were invalidated by the different anastomotic techniques used for the two modalities.

Laser tissue welding

Laser light causes a local heating effect when absorbed by the tissue to which it is applied, and it is on this principle that laser welding relies. The degree and depth of heating, and therefore its tissue effect (Table 13.2) depends on a number of variables (Table 13.3), many of which can be manipulated. The precise mechanism of laser welding is disputed, but the most likely explanations include:

1 Alteration in the periodicity of collagen fibrils resulting in interdigitation, degradation or cross-linking of extracellular matrix proteins.

2 Temperature-dependent denaturation of surface proteins to produce an adhesive coagulum.

3 The production of oxygen radicals, which have been shown to induce polypeptide cross-linkage [18].

Table 13.2 Characteristics and tissue effects of commonly used lasers [16,17].

Laser	Wavelength (nm)	Depth of penetration (mm)	Delivery system	Clinical application
CO_2	10 600	0.019	Articulated arm	Cutting, tissue welding
Argon	458–515	0.3	Fibre	Superficial coagulation, tissue welding
KTP	532	0.8	Fibre	Cutting, coagulation, tissue welding
Dye	400–700	5.1	Fibre	Photodynamic therapy (PDT), laser lithotripsy
Nd : YAG	1064	10	Fibre	Cutting, deep coagulation, ablation, tissue welding

Table 13.3 Factors affecting success of a laser weld.

Tissue factors	Laser parameters
Tissue apposition	Wavelength
Avoidance of tension	Power density
Optical characteristics of tissue	Firing mode
Temperature of weld	Adjuncts

The potential advantages of laser welding are summarized in Table 13.4.

Temperature of the weld

Both excessive and insufficient heating of tissue edges will result in a weak tissue weld. The end-point of laser welding has traditionally been taken as the point at which the tissues shrink and blanch, but before charring. The subjectivity of appreciating this point, and the variable results as a consequence of this subjectivity, have prompted Klioze and colleagues to produce a real-time thermal control system for laser welding, which consists of a remote infra-red sensor and a laser, together with a microcomputer which links the two and automatically limits the laser energy applied to the tissue by shutting off the laser once the preset temperature has been reached. This instrument is still in the prototype phase, but initial results appear to be encouraging [18].

Firing mode

Lasers can be fired in either continuous or pulsed modes—the latter facility allows the pulse length to be kept within the thermal relaxation time of the tissue (a measure of how fast heat is conducted from the target tissue to the surrounding tissues), and so minimizes thermal damage.

Power density

The power density is the total laser energy applied divided by the spot size, and is expressed in watts per square centimetre (W/cm^2). It decreases as the distance between the laser delivery device and its target increases.

Adjuncts

SOLDERS

The use of a protein solder as an adjunct to laser tissue-welding was first described by Poppas, who demonstrated superior results using an egg albumin solder in conjunction with a pulsed milliwatt carbon dioxide (CO_2) laser for the closure of rat urethra, in terms of a 0% fistula rate, compared with 16.8% for laser alone [19]. In the same year, Ganesan and colleagues reported that the addition of an egg albumin solder resulted in a significantly increased success rate and decreased operating time for CO_2 laser-welded patch urethroplasty in rats [20]. It seems that

Table 13.4 Advantages of laser tissue welding.

Energy delivered to a specified area with great precision and without contact
Reduced tissue handling and trauma
Reduced operating time [26]
Avoidance of implanting a foreign body

denaturation of the protein solder occurs when it is heated by exposure to laser light, to form an adhesive coagulum. In a more recent study, Poppas and colleagues demonstrated that the addition of an egg albumin solder for laser-welded closure of rat urethra produced an anastomosis with an immediate bursting strength similar to laser alone, but with a reduced stricture rate: 4.2% with solder compared with 14% for laser alone [21]. The authors hypothesized that the protein solder might also act as a heat sink, decreasing peripheral anastomotic thermal damage. Bass has found that the use of bicomponent protein solders, such as albumin/hyaluronate, albumin/dextran and collagen/hyaluronate is capable of increasing the tensile strength of laser-welded anastomoses by up to 5.3 times that of non-soldered controls [22].

CHROMOPHORES

The use of laser light-absorbing chromophores, whose peak absorption approximate to the wavelength of laser light used, has also been explored: fluorescein isothiocyanate (FITC—480nm) and the potassium–titanyl–phosphate (KTP) laser (532nm); indocyanine green (805nm) and the diode laser (808nm); and India ink (theoretically, electromagnetic radiation of all wavelengths) and the neodymium–yttrium–aluminium–garnet (Nd:YAG) laser (1064nm). Chromophores may also help to reduce peripheral tissue damage by increasing surface laser light absorption. The chromophores may be used either alone or in combination with a protein solder (Fig. 13.5).

A study of laser welding of rabbit aorta using an argon laser (457–514nm) with and without FITC demonstrated that a lower power (3.8W/cm²) was needed for the weld when the aorta was painted with FITC, than without (7.6W/cm²), although this was not statistically significant [23]. A further study of laser welding of canine ureters using the KTP laser, in conjunction with human albumin alone or in conjunction with either iron oxide or FITC, suggests that the weld is stronger in terms of immediate bursting strength if a chromophore is used with an albumin solder, when similar total laser energies were used for the

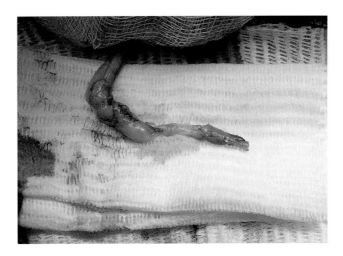

Fig. 13.5 Experimental laser-welded ureteroureterostomy using KTP laser and a fluorescein-doped albumin solder.

various welds [24]. Similar conclusions were drawn from a rabbit study which compared the bursting strength of two-layered sutured colonic anastomoses with those which had been coated with indocyanine green-doped fibrinogen and then irradiated with an 808-nm diode laser [25]. Although the immediate bursting strength was significantly higher in the laser/dye/soldered anastomoses, the differences between the two groups decreased progressively with time.

Choice of laser for tissue welding

Several lasers are suitable for tissue welding (Table 13.2). Results of the use of the CO_2 laser for microsurgical vascular anastomosis have shown that only a superficial weld is produced [26], with sparing of the intima. This is predictable, since CO_2 laser light is strongly absorbed by surface water. The superficiality of the weld is probably also responsible for the high incidence of sperm granulomas seen after CO_2 laser-welded vasovasostomy [27]. The CO_2 laser additionally suffers from the disadvantage that its wavelength precludes transmission via a fibreoptic bundle, rendering it unsuitable for endoscopic use. In contrast, the flexible fibreoptic delivery systems of the argon, KTP and Nd:YAG devices make them ideal for endoscopic application. Compared with the CO_2 laser, these lasers are much more dependent on the optical properties of the tissues upon which they are aimed, as less of their energy is absorbed by surface water. Whatever the choice of laser, the power density needed to accomplish a tissue weld is small relative to the maximum output capacity of most lasers, and well within the capacity of the cheaper and more portable milliwatt diode lasers based on solid-state semiconductor technology.

Laparoscopic application of laser tissue-welding

There are no published reports of the laparoscopic use of laser tissue-welding, although this modality appears to have potential in low-pressure systems, such as the renal tract, biliary tree and small blood vessels.

The author's comparative study of tissue approximation techniques for laparoscopy

The author has recently completed the first comparative study of tissue approximation techniques for laparoscopy, in two phases. In the first phase gelatin resorcin glue (GRF), fibrin glue and KTP laser tissue-welding with a fluorescein-doped 40% human albumin solder, were compared in an open porcine ureteric re-anastomosis model. In the second phase, the best technique from phase I was compared with interrupted 4/0 polyglactin 910 sutures in a retroperitoneoscopic dismembered pyeloplasty model. Assessment criteria for both phases were acute (leak pressure) and chronic (operating time, comparison of pre- and post-operative Whitaker tests, light microscopy and scanning electron microscopy at 6 weeks).

The results are summarized in Table 13.5. In phase I ERF-glued anastomes were insufficiently robust to tolerate rotation of the anastomis, resulting in dehisence on each occasion. This modality was therefore abandoned at this stage. Fibrin glue proved equal to laser welding with respect to leak pressure and change in Whitaker test pressures after 6 weeks, but superior with regard to operating time, and light and electron microscopic appearances, and was therefore selected for comparison with sutured controls in phase II. In this second phase, there was no difference between fibrin-glued and sutured anastomoses with respect to change in Whitaker test pressures, but the fibrin-glued group performed significantly better as regards leak pressure, operating time and both light- and electron- microscopic appearances (Figs 13.6 and 13.7).

Of note, the leak pressures (defined as the pressure at which methylene blue was first seen outside the anastomosis) of the sutured anastomoses in phase II were all within the physiological range for the ureter. In fact,

Table 13.5 Summary of results of comparative study of tissue approximation techniques for laparoscopy by author.

Modality	Median leak pressure with range (mmHg)	Median operating time with range (minutes)	Median change in max. Whitaker test pressure with range (cmH$_2$O)	Light microscopy	Scanning electron microscopy
Phase I					
GRF glue	0 (see text)	–	–	–	–
(*n*=4)					
Fibrin glue	69.2	85	–4.0	Superior appearance	Superior appearance
(*n*=6)	(55–94)	(75–90)	(–11 to +2)		
KTP laser	70.7	134	+7.5	Inferior appearance	Inferior appearance
(*n*=6)	(42–100)	(75–160)	(–8 to +39)		
P*	0.91	0.02	0.30		
Phase II					
Fibrin glue	49.7	142	+5.0	Superior appearance	Superior appearance
(*n*=3)	(48–51)	(130–150)	(–3 to +24†)		
Sutures	8.3	193	–1.0	Inferior appearance	Inferior appearance
(*n*=3)	(4–17)	(150–220)	(–3 to +4)		
P*	0.01	0.01	0.51		

*Mann–Whitney *U*-test.
†Double-pigtail stent displaced to bladder.

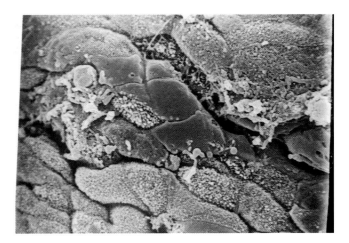

Fig. 13.6 Scanning electron micrograph of experimental fibrin-glued pelviureteric anastomosis after 6 weeks (original magnification ×1800).

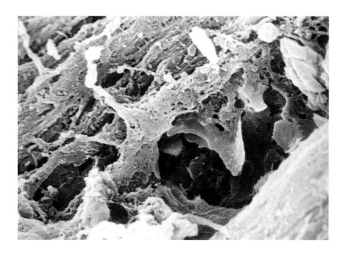

Fig. 13.7 Scanning electron micrograph of experimental sutured pelviureteric anastomosis after 6 weeks (original magnification ×1440).

methylene blue was seen to leak from the suture holes, rather than the anastomotic margin itself, at these pressures. This suggests that urine or bile leakage from sutured anastomoses (conservatively estimated by Persky at 68% following pyeloplasty [28]) is inevitable and may help to explain, at least in part, the phenomenon of anastomotic stricture formation [29].

References

1 Weissberg D, Goetz RH. Necrosis of arterial wall following application of methyl 2-cyanoacrylate. *Surg Gynecol Obstet* 1964; 119: 1248–1252.

2 Dutton J, Yates PO. An experimental study of the effects of a plastic adhesive, methyl 2-cyanoacrylate monomer (M 2 C-1) in various tissues. *J Neurosurg* 1966; 24: 876–882.

3 Brunwald NS, Gay W, Tatooles CJ. Evaluation of cross-linked gelatin as a tissue adhesive and hemostatic agent. Experimental study. *Surgery* 1966; 59: 1024–1030.

4 Chmielewski GW, Saxe JM, Dulchavsky SA, Diebel LN, Bailey JK. Fibrin gel limits intra-abdominal adhesion formation. *Am Surg* 1992; 58: 590–592.

5 Turowski G, Schaadt M, Barthels M, Diehl V, Poliwoda H. Unterschiedlicher Einfluß von Fibrinogen und Faktor XIII auf das Wachstum von Primar—und Kulturfibroblasten. In: Schimpf Kl, ed. *Fibrin, Fibrinogen und Fibrinkleber.* Stuttgart: F K Schattauer Verlag, 1980: 227–237.

6 Durham LH, Willatt DJ, Yung MW, Jones I, Stevenson PA, Ramadan MF. A method for preparation of fibrin glue. *J Laryngol Otol* 1987; 101: 1182–1186.

7 Kram HB, Garces MA, Klein SR, Shoemaker WC. Common bile duct anastomosis using fibrin glue. *Arch Surg* 1985; 120: 1250–1256.

8 Holmes SAV, James M, Whitfield HN. Potential use of tissue adhesive in urinary tract surgery. *Br J Urol* 1992; 69: 647–650.

9 Niederberger C, Ross LS, Mackenzie B, Schacht MJ, Cho Y. Vasovasostomy in rabbits using fibrin adhesive prepared from a single human source. *J Urol* 1993; 149: 183–185.

10 Ball RA, Steinberg J, Wilson LA, Loughlin KR. Comparison of

vasovasostomy techniques in rats utilizing conventional microsurgical suture, carbon dioxide laser, and fibrin tissue adhesives. *Urology* 1993; 41: 479–483.

11 Byrne DJ, Hardy J, Wood RAB, McIntosh R, Hopwood D, Cuschieri A. Adverse influence of fibrin sealant on the healing of high-risk sutured colonic anastomoses. *J Roy Coll Surg Edinb* 1992; 37: 394–398.

12 van der Ham AC, Kort WJ, Weijma M, van den Ingh HFGM, Jeekel J. Effect of fibrin sealant on the healing of colonic anastomosis in the rat. *Br J Surg* 1991; 78: 49–53.

13 Houston KA, Rotstein OD. Fibrin sealant in high-risk colonic anastomoses. *Arch Surg* 1988; 123: 230–234.

14 Byrne DJ, Hardy J, Wood RAB, McIntosh R, Cuschieri A. Effect of fibrin glues on the mechanical properties of healing wounds. *Br J Surg* 1991; 78: 841–843.

15 McKay TC, Albala DM, Gehrin BE, Castelli M. Laparoscopic ureteral reanastomosis using fibrin glue. *J Urol* 1994; 152: 1637–1640.

16 Jacques SL. Laser–tissue interactions: photochemical, photothermal and photomechanical. *Surg Clin North Am* 1992; 72: 531–558.

17 McNicholas TA. A practical guide to laser treatment. In: McNicholas TA, ed. *Lasers in Urology.* New York: Springer Verlag, 1990: 23–39.

18 Klioze SD, Poppas DP, Rooke CT, Choma TJ, Schlossberg SM. Development and initial application of a real time thermal control system for laser tissue welding. *J Urol* 1994; 52: 744–748.

19 Poppas DP, Schlossberg SM, Richmond IL, Gilbert DA, Devine CJ. Laser welding in urethral surgery: improved results with a protein solder. *J Urol* 1988; 139: 415–417.

20 Ganesan GS, Poppas DP, Devine CJ, Schlossberg SM. Urethral reconstruction using the carbon dioxide laser: an experimental evaluation. *J Urol* 1989; 142: 1139–1141.

21 Poppas DP, Rooke CT, Schlossberg SM. Optical parameters for CO_2 laser reconstruction of urethral tissue using a protein solder. *J Urol* 1992; 148: 220–224.

22 Bass LS. New solders for laser welding and sealing. *Lasers Med Surg* 1993; Suppl. 5: 63.

23 Chuck RS, Oz MC, Delohery TM *et al.* Dye-enhanced laser tissue welding. *Lasers Surg Med* 1989; 9: 471–477.

24 Poppas DP, Sutaria P, Sosa RE, Miniberg DT, Vaughan ED, Schlossberg SM. Re-establishing continuity of the ureter using laser tissue welding techniques: evaluation of new laser tissue welding solders for laparoscopic surgery. *J Urol* 1992; 148: 244.

25 Moazami N, Oz MC, Bass LS, Treat MR. Reinforcement of colonic anastomoses with a laser and dye-enhanced fibrinogen. *Arch Surg* 1990; 125: 1452–1454.

26 Neblett CR, Morris JR, Thomsen S. Laser-assisted microsurgical anastomosis. *Neurosurgery* 1986; 19: 914–934.

27 Jarrow JP, Cooley BC, Marshall FF. Laser assisted vasal anastomosis in the rat and man. *J Urol* 1986; 36: 1132–1135.

28 Persky L, McDougal WS, Kedia K. Management of initial pyeloplasty failure. *J Urol* 1981; 125: 695–697.

29 Keetch D, Andriole GL, Catalona WJ. Complications of radical retropubic prostatectomy. *AUA Update Series* 1994; 13: 46–51.

14 Pyeloplasty

C. G. EDEN

Although dismembered pyeloplasty, as originally described by Anderson and Hynes in 1949 [1], is associated with the best long-term results for the treatment of pelviureteric junction (PUJ) obstruction (Table 14.1), the loin incision necessary to perform it results in significant post-operative wound discomfort [2], prolonged hospitalization [2] and a 6–12-week period before normal activities can be resumed. Predictably, therefore, minimal access techniques for the correction of PUJ obstruction have attracted considerable interest. Despite encouraging early results (Table 14.2) the benefits of balloon dilatation of the PUJ are not durable [12,13], except following the early treatment of post-surgical anastomotic strictures. In expert hands, endopyelotomy fares much better: a review of the results of the major series of endopyelotomy (Table 14.3) and open pyeloplasty shows that the best attainable success rate for endopyelotomy

Table 14.1 Results of open dismembered pyeloplasty.

Author	No. units	Age range	Min. follow-up (months)	Success rate (%)	Criteria*
Graversen et al. (1987) [3]	52	0–41 years	12	85	S/I/B
Guys et al. (1988) [4]	50	0–7 months	6	90	R
King et al. (1984) [5]	11	3–10 days	3	100	I/R
Mikkelsen et al. (1992) [6]	21	11–72 years	44	94	I
Nguyen et al. (1989) [7]	68	2 days–28 years	36	94	I/R
O'Reilly (1989) [8]	30	5–64 years	6	73	R
Poulsen et al. (1987) [9]	35	3–69 years	12	93	I/R
Sommer et al. (1989) [10]	22	6–75 years	12	75	S
Wolpert et al. (1989) [11]	114	Infants and children	6	90	I/R

*S, symptoms; I, intravenous urography; B, biochemistry; R, renography.

Table 14.2 Results of balloon dilatation of the pelviureteric junction.

Author	No. units	Age range	Min. follow-up (months)	Success rate (%)	Criteria*
O'Flynn et al. (1989) [12]	31	18–70	3	68	R
McClinton et al. (1993) [13]	49	17–83	3	78	R

*R, renography.

Table 14.3 Results of endopyelotomy.

Author	No. units	Age range (years)	Min. follow-up (months)	Success rate (%)	Criteria*
Badlani et al. (1986) [14]	31	7–79	6	87	I
Brannen et al. (1988) [15]	10	19–76	3	80	I
Karlin and Smith (1988) [16]	73	Not stated	3	89	I/R
Korth et al. (1988) [17]	71	15–79	6	79	I
Motola et al. (1993) [18]	212	2–84	6	86	I
Naito et al. (1991) [19]	14	13–56	6	86	I
Payne et al. (1988) [20]	20	Not stated	12	60	R
Perez et al. (1992) [21]	17	15–69	4	88	I
Ramsay et al. (1984) [22]	28	15–72	9	64	I/R
van Cangh et al. (1994) [23]	102	Not stated	12	73	I/R/S

*I, intravenous urography; R, renography; S, symptoms.

lags only 10% behind that of its open counterpart [14–23]. In fact this figure of 10% is an overestimate, since nearly all series of endopyelotomy exclude patients with a large renal pelvis and those cases in which there is circumstantial evidence of a crossing lower pole vessel at the PUJ. Endopyelotomy also suffers from the disadvantage that when it is performed by the least invasive (retrograde) route, it is associated with a ureteric stricture rate of up to 20% [24].

A retroperitoneoscopic approach to dismembered pyeloplasty promises to combine the best surgical procedure for the correction of PUJ reconstruction with the least traumatic method of access, and should, in theory, give the patient the very best long-term result in terms of anastomotic patency, combined with the minimum of morbidity. A comparative experimental study of tissue approximation techniques by the author (see Chapter 13) has confirmed the feasibility of this approach and suggests that the lengthy operating times previously reported for this procedure [25] might be reduced by the use of fibrin glue, and the long-term anastomotic patency rate might be improved yet further by reducing peri-anastomotic urine extravasation and the extent of the inflammatory reaction at the anastomosis.

Operative details

The patient is submitted to a general anaesthetic with muscle relaxation and endotracheal intubation. An appropriate parenteral antibiotic is administered prior to cystoscopy and insertion of a double-pigtail ureteric stent under fluoroscopy. A urethral catheter is then inserted.

Access

With the patient in the full lateral position and the operating table fully broken, a 2-cm transverse incision is made immediately anterior to the tip of the twelfth rib. The incision is deepened with scissor dissection and the three muscle layers of the anterior abdominal wall successively split until

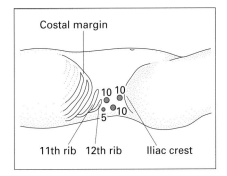

Fig. 14.1 Port placement for retroperitoneoscopic pyeloplasty. Port diameters in millimetres.

the thoracolumbar fascia is encountered. This is incised to enter the retroperitoneum, carefully avoiding the subcostal neurovascular bundle. The author makes no attempt to dissect deep to Gerota's fascia at this stage, as he has found that placement of the balloon dissector outside this layer results in a larger initial workspace. Accordingly, a Helmstein balloon (see Fig. 1.5) is inserted into the retroperitoneum and the balloon gradually inflated with 0.5–0.7 litres of air, depending on the size of the patient, using the rubber bulb of a sphygmomanometer. The balloon is kept inflated at this volume for 5 minutes to tamponade any septal vessels which might otherwise bleed, and is then removed. Ports are then inserted (Fig. 14.1) under guidance of a finger inserted into the retroperitoneum. This precaution minimizes the risk of lacerating the peritoneum and is more expedient than port insertion under endoscopic control. The camera port (without trocar) is inserted through the initial skin incision, which is sealed around it using Allis forceps or a heavy purse-string suture. The carbon dioxide gas supply is connected to a non-camera port (to minimize cooling and misting of the laparoscope) and the warmed laparoscope inserted to inspect the cavity.

Pyeloplasty

An inadequate retroperitoneal workspace should be enlarged with blunt dissection. Gerota's fascia is incised, and the stented ureter is identified at the lower pole of the kidney and mobilized towards the pelviureteric segment, taking care to preserve the upper peri-ureteric vessels. A 2/0 nylon suture inserted percutaneously, passed under the ureter (Fig. 14.2) and back through the skin, frees both hand instruments for the important proximal dissection. Difficulty at this stage is always due to inadequate (or lack of) incision of Gerota's fascia, without which neither the kidney nor the ureter can be identified or dissected. Dissection of the lower pole and lateral border of the kidney allows it to be rotated anteromedially and held in this position using a fan retractor (United States Surgical Corporation, Norwalk, Connecticut, USA) inserted through the most

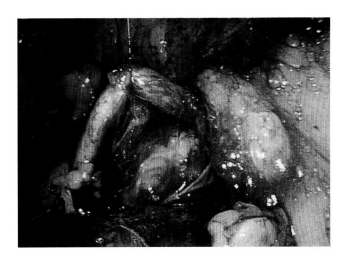

Fig. 14.2 A percutaneous nylon traction suture lifting the ureter at the lower pole of the kidney.

caudal 10-mm port. Once the renal pelvis has been totally dissected (Fig. 14.3) the limits of the reduction pyeloplasty are planned. The author has not found the insertion of stay sutures to be helpful or necessary.

The ureter is carefully divided just below the PUJ, taking care not to damage the ureteric stent (Fig. 14.4), which is retrieved from the pelvis. The lateral aspect of the divided ureter is then grasped with fine curved forceps and the ureter spatulated over 2 cm on the opposite side (Fig. 14.5). Redundant pelvic tissue, including the PUJ, is excised (Fig. 14.6). The first suture (the author's preference is for 4/0 polyglactin 910 (Ethicon, Edinburgh, UK) mounted on a round-bodied 20-mm curved needle) is inserted at the most dependent part of the anastomosis (Fig. 14.7), and the superior coil of the double-pigtail stent is replaced into the renal pelvis. The medial aspect (Fig. 14.8) and then the lateral aspect (Fig. 14.9) of the anastomosis is approximated using just sufficient interrupted sutures to appose the urothelium, working towards the proximal lip of the anastomosis. All knots are tied intracorporeally with three opposed half-hitches.

Solutions of (i) calcium chloride and thrombin (500 international units per millilitre), and (ii) fibrin and aprotinin (Tisseel™; Immuno, Vienna, Austria) are warmed to 37°C using the manufacturer's purpose-designed

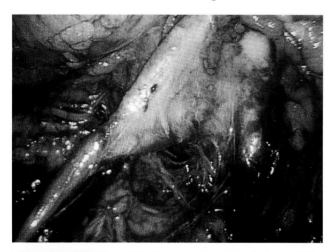

Fig. 14.3 Dissected pelviureteric segment.

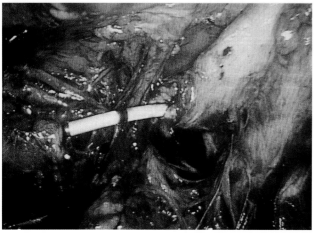

Fig. 14.4 Pelviureteric junction dismembered over a 6F double-pigtail catheter.

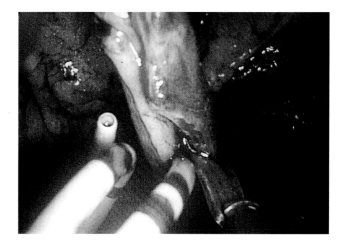

Fig. 14.5 Spatulation of the ureter.

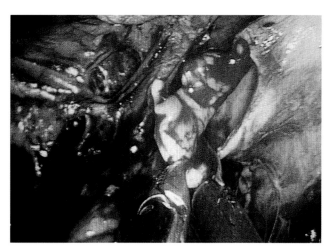

Fig. 14.6 Open renal pelvis following excision of redundant pelvic tissue.

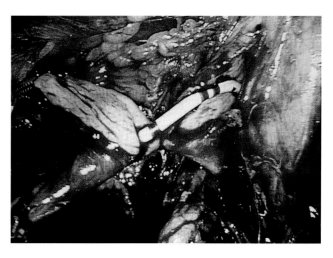

Fig. 14.7 The first suture has been inserted at the most dependent part of the anastomosis.

electrical warmer, before being loaded into separate syringes; this arrangement allows delivery of a 1:1 mixture of the solutions via a double-lumen flexible catheter inserted percutaneously through a 12G cannula under endoscopic vision. The rapidly polymerizing fibrin glue is then used to

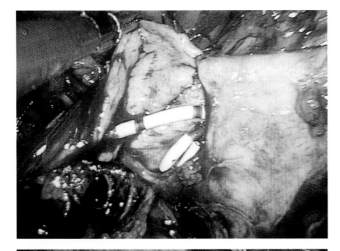

Fig. 14.8 Approximation of the medial aspect of the pyeloplasty.

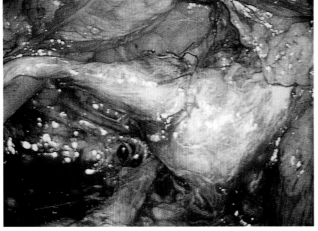

Fig. 14.9 Appearance of the anastomosis following insertion of sutures.

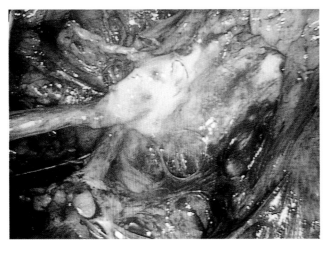

Fig. 14.10 Completed anastomosis following the application of fibrin glue.

coat both sides of the reconstructed PUJ (Fig. 14.10). A tube drain is inserted through the most caudal port and laid along the lateral surface of the kidney under endoscopic control. All wounds are closed using a 0 polyglactin 910 fascial suture and a 2/0 polyglactin 910 subcuticular suture. The wounds are infiltrated with local anaesthetic and a diclofenac sodium suppository inserted, unless there is a specific contraindication.

Post-operative care

The urinary catheter may be removed the following morning, together with the wound drain. Free fluids by mouth are usually tolerated on the first post-operative morning and a full diet by the end of the day. The double-pigtail ureteric catheter is removed using a flexible cystoscope at 6 weeks.

Results

At the time of writing, the author has successfully completed eight of nine attempted cases, the results of which are summarized in Table 14.4. In the single failure, although it was possible to dissect and dismember the PUJ, spatulate the ureter and tailor the pelvis, it was not possible to reapproximate the shortened fibrotic ureter to the renal pelvis without tension either laparoscopically or at open surgery, necessitating interposition of the appendix. Biopsy of the ureter revealed retroperitoneal fibrosis.

The mean operating time (first skin incision to closure of the last port site) of 185 minutes compares very favourably with the mean operating time of 355 minutes for the six patients in the literature who have undergone transperitoneal laparoscopic pyeloplasty [27,28], and 380 minutes for the two patients who have undergone retroperitoneoscopic pyeloplasty [25]. This reduction in operating time is likely to be due to a combination of the following factors:

1 Less tissue dissection is necessary to gain access to the kidney using a retroperitoneal endoscopic approach.

2 Direct access to the pelviureteric segment is obtained using this approach, which is unobscured by loops of bowel.

3 The use of fibrin glue necessitates the placement of fewer sutures than a conventionally sutured pyeloplasty. The use of fibrin glue also minimizes anastomotic urine leakage, which is confirmed by the fact that the drain

Table 14.4 Summary of results of author's clinical series.

Patient no.	Sex	Age	Weight (kg)	Operating time (minutes)	Opiate analgesic requirement (mg morphine sulphate i.m.)	Post-operative hospitalization (nights)	Diuretic MAG3 excretion curve at 3 months [26]
1	F	49	64	230	40	4	1
2	F	51	60	Opened at 120 min	80	14	3a
3	M	34	91	170	0	2	1
4	F	21	52	150	0	2	3a
5	M	17	68	210	10	3	2*
6	M	59	76	210	0	2	3a
7	M	42	100	180	0	2	2*
8	M	46	62	180	0	2	Not available
9	M	60	82	150	0	2	Not available
Mean*		41.0	74.4	185	6.2	2.4	
Mode		–	–	–	0	2	

*Excludes patient no. 2.

could be removed within the first 14 hours following pyeloplasty in all patients.

The short period of post-operative hospitalization (mode = two nights) and low parenteral opiate requirement (mode = 0 mg morphine sulphate) reflect the absence of the significant degree of patient discomfort which is typical following open pyeloplasty via a loin incision, and which may become a protracted problem.

Comparison of these results with a contemporaneous series of ten patients (Table 14.5), who were well-matched for age and weight ($P = 0.46$ and 0.34, respectively; two-sample t-test), undergoing open pyeloplasty by the authors at an affiliated institution, demonstrates

Table 14.5 Summary of results of contemporaneous series of open pyeloplasty at author's institution.

Patient no.	Age	Weight (kg)	Opiate analgesic requirement (mg morphine sulphate i.m.)	Post-operative hospitalization (nights)	Complications
1	32	69	80	7	
2	72	65	90	27	Wound infection; deep venous thrombosis
3	61	75	80	11	
4	74	63	30	12	
5	20	66	60	6	Infected urinoma
6	53	64	30	7	
7	26	82	10	6	
8	50	47	40	9	
9	74	55	50	8	
10	19	90	40	10	
Mean	48.1	67.6	51	10.3	

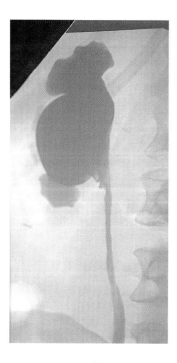

Fig. 14.11 Retrograde ureteropyelogram of patient number 7 (see Table 14.4) 6 months following surgery demonstrating a patent pelviureteric anastomosis.

a significantly reduced post-operative opiate analgesic requirement ($P = 0.0004$; two-sample t-test) and shorter post-operative hospitalization ($P = 0.003$; two-sample t-test) in the endoscopic group. Two serious infective complications requiring drainage were noted in the open group, one of which was further complicated by a radiologically proven deep venous thrombosis. In contrast, no post-operative complications were noted in the endoscopic group.

Diuresis renographic follow-up at one year demonstrates unobstructed upper tract drainage in six of the eight successfully operated cases. Although the remaining two renal units (which contributed 33% and 18% of total renal function) produced a rising curve on both F+15 and F-15 diuresis MAG3 renography, subsequent retrograde ureteropyelography demonstrated that contrast in the pelvis rapidly drained into the ureter when the patient was turned prone in each case (Fig. 14.11), indicating that pooling of the radioisotope in the dilated pelvicalyceal system of a poorly functioning kidney had produced a false positive result.

Although longer-term renographic follow-up is needed to determine the true clinical utility of this technique, the initial results give reason for optimism.

References

1 Anderson JC, Hynes W. Retrocaval ureter. A case diagnosed pre-operatively and treated successfully by a plastic operation. *Br J Urol* 1949; 21: 209–214.

2 Eden CG, Carter PG, Haigh AC, Sherwood RA, Green DW, Coptcoat MJ. The metabolic response to laparoscopic and open nephrectomy. *Min Invas Ther* 1994; 3: 43–50.

3 Graversen HP, Tofte T, Genster HG. Uretero-Pelvic stenosis. *Int Urol Nephrol* 1987; 19: 245–251.

4 Guys JM, Borella F, Monfort G. Ureteropelvic junction obstructions: prenatal diagnosis and neonatal surgery in 47 cases. *J Pediatr Surg* 1988; 23: 156–158.

5 King LR, Coughlin PWF, Bloch EC, Bowie JD, Ansong K, Hanna MK. The case for immediate pyeloplasty in the neonate with ureteropelvic junction obstruction. *J Urol* 1984; 132: 725–728.

6 Mikkelsen SS, Rasmussen BS, Jensen TM, Hanghoj-Petersen W, Christensen PO. Long-term follow-up of patients with hydronephrosis treated by Anderson–Hynes pyeloplasty. *Br J Urol* 1992; 79: 121–124.

7 Nguyen DH, Aliabadi H, Ercole CJ, Gonzalez R. Nonintubated Anderson–Hynes repair of ureteropelvic junction obstruction in 60 patients. *J Urol* 1989; 142: 704–706.

8 O'Reilly PH. Functional outcome of pyeloplasty for ureteropelvic junction obstruction: prospective study in 30 consecutive cases. *J Urol* 1989; 142: 273–276.

9 Poulsen EU, Frokjaer J, Taagehoj-Jensen F *et al*. Diuresis renography and simultaneous renal pelvic pressure in hydronephrosis. *J Urol* 1987; 138: 272–275.

10 Sommer P, Lyngdorf P, Frimodt-Moller C. Late results of pyeloplasty by the Anderson–Hynes method. *Int Urol Nephrol* 1989; 21: 139–144.

11 Wolpert JJ, Woodard JR, Parrott TS. Pyeloplasty in the young infant. *J Urol* 1989; 142: 573–575.

12 O'Flynn KO, Hehir M, McKelvie G, Hussey J, Steyn J. Endoballoon rupture and stenting for pelviureteric junction obstruction: technique and early results. *Br J Urol* 1989; 64: 572–574.

13 McClinton S, Steyn JH, Hussey JK. Retrograde balloon dilatation for pelviureteric junction obstruction. *Br J Urol* 1993; 71: 152–155.

14 Badlani G, Eshghi M, Smith AD. Percutaneous surgery for ureteropelvic junction obstruction (endopyelotomy): technique and early results. *J Urol* 1986; 135: 26–28.

15 Brannen GE, Bush WH, Lewis GP. Endopyelotomy for primary repair of ureteropelvic junction obstruction. *J Urol* 1988; 139: 29–32.

16 Karlin GS, Smith AD. Endopyelotomy. *Urol Clin North Am* 1988; 15: 439–444.

17 Korth K, Kuenkel M, Erschig M. Percutaneous pyeloplasty. *Urology* 1988; 31: 503–509.

18 Motola JA, Badlani GH, Smith AD. Results of 212 consecutive endopyelotomies: an 8-year followup. *J Urol* 1993; 149: 453–456.

19 Naito S, Yamaguchi A, Tanaka M *et al.* Endopyelotomy for treatment of ureteropelvic junction obstruction. *Urol Int* 1991; 46: 309–312.

20 Payne SR, Coptcoat MJ, Kellett MJ, Wickham JEA. Effective intubation for percutaneous pyelolysis. *Eur Urol* 1988; 14: 477–481.

21 Perez LM, Friedman RM, Carson III, CC. Endoureteropyelotomy in adults. *Urology* 1992; 39: 71–76.

22 Ramsay JWA, Miller RA, Kellett MJ, Blackford HN, Wickham JEA, Whitfield HN. Percutaneous pyelolysis. *Br J Urol* 1984; 56: 586–588.

23 van Cangh PJ, Wilmart JF, Opsomer RJ, Abi-Aad A, Wese FX, Lorge F. Long-term results and late recurrence after endoureteropyelotomy: a critical analysis of prognostic factors. *J Urol* 1994; 151: 934–937.

24 Meretyk I, Meretyk S, Clayman RV. Endopyelotomy: comparison of ureteroscopic retrograde and antegrade percutaneous techniques. *J Urol* 1992; 148: 775–783.

25 Rassweiler JJ, Hemkel TO, Stock C, Alken P. Retroperitoneoscopic surgery—technique, indications and first experience. *Min Invas Ther* 1994; 3: 179–195.

26 Lupton EW, Testa HJ, O'Reilly PH *et al.* Diuresis renography and morphology in upper urinary tract obstruction. *Br J Urol* 1979; 51: 10–14.

27 Schuessler WW, Grune MT, Tecuanhuey LV, Preminger GM. Laparoscopic dismembered pyeloplasty. *J Urol* 1993; 150: 1795–1799.

28 Kavoussi LR, Peters CA. Laparoscopic pyeloplasty. *J Urol* 1993; 150: 1891–1894.

Index